LUMINOUS ESSENCE

LUMINOUS ESSENCE

NEW LIGHT ON THE HEALING BODY

AN ALTERNATIVE HEALER'S STORY

DANIEL SANTOS, D.O.M.

A publication supported by
THE KERN FOUNDATION

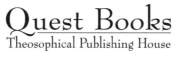

Quest Books
Theosophical Publishing House

Wheaton, Illinois ◆ Madras, India

The Theosophical Publishing House
P.O. Box 270
Wheaton, IL 60189-0270

A publication of the Theosophical Publishing House,
a department of the Theosophical Society in America

Library of Congress Cataloging-in-Publication Data

Santos, Daniel, D.O.M.
   Luminous essence: new light on the healing body, an alternative healer's
story / Daniel Santos. — 1st Quest ed.
      p.   cm.
   Originally published: Santa Fe, N.M.: Luminous Press, 1994.
   ISBN 0-8356-0755-0
   1. New Age movement.   2. Alternative medicine—Philosophy.
3. Santos, Daniel, D.O.M.   4. Healers—United States.   I. Title.
BP605.N48S25   1997
615.5—DC21   97-4460
                                                                   CIP

Copyright acknowledgment for excerpts:
Thomas Merton: *The Way of Chuang-Tzu*. Copyright c1965 by The Abbey of
Gethsemani. Reprinted by permission of New Directions Publishing Corp.
World rights.
Chuang Tsu. Copyright c1974 by Feng and English. Translation by Feng and
English. Reprinted by permission of Alfred A. Knopf, Inc.
Tsu Tao Te Ching. Copyright c1974 by Feng and English. Translation by Feng
and English. Reprinted by permission of Alfred A. Knopf, Inc.

6   5   4   3   2   1   *   97   98   99   00   01   02

Printed in the United States of America

CONTENTS

ACKNOWLEDGMENTS

I would like to thank Rhoshel Lenroot for helping me with this book in the initial stages and Andrew Elliott for helping to organize and get this material ready for print. I would particularly like to thank Joseph Durepos, my agent, and Brenda Rosen, my editor. Brenda was a great help in reorganizing my material to more fully and clearly focus the ideas in this book.

I would also like to express deepest gratitude and appreciation to all of my teachers.

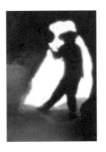

INTRODUCTION

The body knows what it is doing. Even as a seed, given time, space, and the right conditions, will grow into a tree, the body, when it can remain in touch with its integrity, will grow into its potential as a human being. This is what I call the "healing body."

When we break a bone, there is an integrity with force and power behind it which knows how to knit that bone. When we cut ourselves, there is a template of how we should or could be that comes to our assistance to mend our wound. There is a luminous essence inside of us at many different levels that embodies our potential.

My name is Daniel Santos. I am a healer. I have practiced acupuncture and other healing arts for almost twenty-five years. I have searched for a real cure. I first saw simple patterns of disease, such as an injured shoulder or pain in the stomach, as isolated events. I believed that these isolated events needed to be cured in and of themselves. Later I began to see interrelationships between these seemingly isolated ailments. I then became aware that disease exists in huge patterns running up and down the body. In studying these bigger patterns and learning about them in my own body, I began to see the body as a web of light—ribbons of light—an iridescent web of creation that we manufacture daily.

In my search for completion, I have been forced to synthesize and understand a great variety of truths. I have been exposed to the teachings of the East, studying in both India and China. I have been deeply moved by the shamanistic perspectives and dreamscapes offered in both Taoism and in the Native American cosmologies of North America, South America, and Mexico.

I have also been exposed to the truths offered in Western science and medicine, and the advantages and limitations of dividing our selves into body, mind, and spirit. In addition, for over twenty-five years, I have studied Asian and shamanistic medicine, including acupuncture and its theoretical predecessors, Chinese yoga and the internal martial arts.

As a result of these experiences, I have been forced to expand my idea of who I am. I realized that within me there is something that knows—my "luminous essence"—and from this I have shaped a new fluid model of reality based on body consciousness.

In *Luminous Essence*, I explain why it is important to view our body as a luminous cell of pressure and talk about how our habitual patterns affect us and how deeply they are implanted in our being. I also explore body consciousness—how our bodies are conditioned by the consensus—and describe a new way to view the body in relation to pressure and gravity. It is because we are on the Earth that we have bodies. Thus, our very experience of our body is based on the Earth's gravity, and it is through gravity that the Earth nurtures and cares for us. I write about how the Earth's gravity creates a pressure in us that increases the circulation in our being. Learning to maximize this pressure by lining up vertically, in terms of heaven and earth, we can establish a basis upon which to create a new experience of human potential.

As children we are taught who we are supposed to be. We

erroneously begin to identify ourselves as the lens through which we learn to perceive rather than as the light that shines through that lens, our luminous essence. By repetitiously experiencing the world in the restricted way in which we have been conditioned, we ignore the vast variety of other ways we could look at ourselves and the world. This limits the amount of our luminous essence that we are able to express and restricts our contact with the world at large.

By the time we are adults, we have fixated our light in the same patterns so many times that those circuits of light have dimmed from overuse. The result is a lack of vitality and, eventually, disease.

Incomplete circulation in our bodies forms patterns. These patterns predispose our bodies to diseases which can shorten our life span. Disease patterns are like cobwebs that develop when the web of light around the body is not energized in its completeness. It is similar to the cobwebs that gather in a corner of a building due to lack of circulation.

This book is about bringing our light back into proper circulation. We can only feel whole and complete when we embody our potential. To do this we must understand both personal and cultural patterns of ill health and how our negative experiences of life are stored in areas of our bodies. We must also understand the manner in which diseases are culturally transmitted through generations.

I chose the narrative form for this book because I love stories. Stories can best convey information that, in reality, is more totally communicated body to body. That is how I learned it and how I would like you to learn it. I like stories because they can allow for a free flowing dialogue, a possibility for the exploration of physical movement, and a container for the expression of contextual cues. I feel that the weaving of a tale based on my real experiences is the optimal way for presenting the multisensual communication that really goes on between bodies.

In my experience as a healer three major areas of focus have made a quantum difference in my being. These are: 1) the study of body mechanics, 2) the study of our psycho-emotional relationships with each other and how these express themselves through our bodies, 3) the study of shamanistic healing, including Eastern medicine, acupuncture, and herbology.

I present this knowledge through the relationship of a student—myself—with his teachers. Two of these, Huang and Esmeralda, were my actual mentors. Eulogio is a composite, based largely on my own experiences as a healer and those healing practioners I have studied under. The body of knowledge is a teacher in and of itself, flowing through time. Thus Eulogio is both myself and the wisdom of the teachings personified. In reflecting on this knowledge and its sources in my life, I have come to appreciate anew that the wisdom of healing is best communicated to the body directly.

In this age of computers and mass communication, we have both the opportunity to take a break from our habituated use of the body and the time to examine the body's potential in a new way. For countless centuries, ways of behaving have been passed physically from body to body, through one generation after another, from grandparents to parents to children.

Humanity is now at a stage where old values and social structures are breaking down. This period of human transition is an important juncture, a time to reassess the nature of being human. In short, when things fall apart, an opening is created for something new. This book is about exploring a new way of being conscious of our bodies. It presents a way in which we can ultimately return to the body as our primary tool of communication.

I hope that the new theory of body consciousness offered in this book will spark realizations in you which will help weave together frayed threads in the tapestry of truth within which you live.

PART ONE

THE LUMINOUS
CELL OF PRESSURE

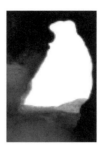

Pressure and Gravity

Our luminous body is the most incredible tool we have. The way we perceive our body is the center post of our perception of reality. Everything radiates outward from this perception. If you change your perception of the body, you can change your perception of reality.

— Huang

H e pushed me again. I went flying across the room one more time. I felt like I had been hit by an electric charge. As I staggered backwards, the world moved slowly. I felt encapsulated in a different flow of time. It was like the feeling you have during an automobile accident. I felt disjointed, yet crystal clear.

"If you had been soft and pliable when I hit you, you would still be standing up," Huang said.

"But then I would have missed this feeling!" I replied.

"You and your feelings, that isn't the point here. What I want you to learn is that you can be soft but strong at the same time. Pliable and resilient. Iron wrapped in silk.

"Now, again: If you had been soft and pliable when I hit you, you would still be standing up! Remember, soft does not mean limp. Soft means sensitive and alive, responsive and strong, connected and powerful. Full of pressure."

I felt like a beginner, like I always did after being around Huang for ten minutes, but I swallowed my embarrassment.

"How can I be soft and hard at the same time?" I asked.

"Well," he said, "if you're too hard, you're not sensitive. I can flow around you like water. You'll never be able to react fast enough.

"If you're limp and open, sensitive without strength and suppleness behind it, you're a sitting duck," he said.

"So how do you do them both together?" I asked in confusion.

"Connect your whole body through pressure. Cut the thoughts and your old ways of acting and reacting. Trust your natural awareness and give strength to it. Let this strength fill you. It knows."

He smiled and motioned to me to come sit beside him. We were in his martial arts studio, one wall letting sunlight pour in from the south, the other walls nestled into the hillside. The air inside was very still. He assured me that it was because we were underground, securely held within the nurturing power of the earth. He told me that down here we could concentrate within ourselves because the air and light that we breathed and moved in was recirculated back to us. If we were outside, we would be in the forces of wind and water much more, receiving energy from the wind and sending it back as part of a greater entity.

He leaned over and touched my shoulder with his hand for a moment.

"The body of the earth is a fluid pressurized mass contained in the luminous cell of its atmosphere. So, too, is the body. The body is a big cell of life, a big sac of tissue. A sac that is full of water. This sac of water is being held down by gravity. This has the effect of creating pressure in the sac of the body and the luminous membrane around it.

"When we relax, truly relax, we allow for the maximum interconnectedness within this sac. Real relaxing is allowing the force of gravity to work on our bodies. When we were babies, we were relaxed in this way.

"When you sleep, you rest. When you rest, you relax. That relaxation allows gravity to pull down on all parts of your body and create pressure and interconnectedness that revitalizes your being.

"Do you have any questions?"

I knew that I had a question, but my thoughts were somewhat unclear, so I asked, "This pressure idea and seeing the body as one big sac is fine, but what about all the bones and muscles and organs in the body?"

He looked at me and smiled.

"We begin life as a single luminous cell. That cell divides into two, but remains connected. It divides into four, eight, sixteen, continually remaining interconnected. Then the organs begin to develop, but looking at it in a larger context, we're still one big sac of water that is interconnected.

"Bones and tendons develop within this sac of tissue, still resonating with the original tissue that they are made from. They are all created from the same substance. So the organs, muscles, and bones are made up of this same interconnectiveness. Fluid is moved by pressure through the sac, providing nourishment to all its parts. I believe that in Western medicine, a somewhat analogous way of seeing this interconnectedness is in the concept of the connective tissue or fascia."

I agreed that this made sense, rather astounded by his ideas of body mechanics.

He smiled again.

"You may have noticed, I used the words: 'moved by pressure.' We can learn to consciously move this pressure through our bodies."

Huang looked out the window.

"The mind moves with this pressure. This pressure is the precursor of light," he said. "But we'll talk more about this later."

Huang then got up and let his arms hang limply at his sides. "This isn't relaxation. This is just limpness. It has no pressure or concentration in it. Most people think of relaxation as being limp."

He gestured to me to join him and raised his limp arm. Then he made a fist, tensing the muscles in his arm.

"Now push down on my arm."

I put my hand on his arm and started pushing down.

"Do it with both hands," he said.

5

Mustering all of his strength, he could not prevent me from bending his arm. He smiled.

"I will now connect my body together with pressure," he said.

He held out his arm. His hand and fingers were very relaxed. I pushed down with both hands. I pushed down harder and harder, to no avail. His arm simply wouldn't move.

"Feel my muscles," he said. I felt them. Much to my surprise, they were soft.

"This is pressure. This is relaxation," he said. "This is lining up with gravity. My whole body is connected with itself." Huang motioned for me to let go of his arm.

"Now you know about pressure," he continued. "You have felt it in my body. Remember, bodies talk to bodies. Your body will remember this after your mind has forgotten."

He repeated this to me five different ways, until he was sure I had memorized, if not grasped, the idea that there is a vibrational transmission or language between bodies.

"We will start to work on how you can retain this same sense of relaxation and interconnectedness while you are moving," he continued. "We can learn to move the pressure throughout our body, through our body motions, such as walking, turning, and falling," he said as, without warning, he pushed me to the floor.

From my position on the ground, I looked up at him and he continued.

"In fact, a useful way to think about how the body works is to see the body as an organic computer. The bulk of the information in this organic computer is kept in the trunk of the body where the organs and bowels are," he said, placing one hand on his chest and the other on his abdomen.

"The head and face make up the screen of this computer. The screen takes the inputs that are coming up from the trunk of the body and displays them. These four limbs are like the cables that plug us into the world," he said, raising his right leg and arm.

"It is through the motions of our shoulders, elbows, hands, hips, knees, and feet that we can move around, feed ourselves, interact with other people, and interface with the world. Pressure is what pushes the energy from our torso, through our extremities, out to our hands and feet.

"In fact, as you know from your work, most of the important acupuncture points are between the knees and toes and the elbows and fingers," he continued. He placed his forearm against his calf to show me how the shoulders and hips, elbows and knees, wrists and ankles are connected to each other.

"There are two reasons for this," he said. "One is that the energy which is mixed together in the trunk of the body is more differentiated in the extremities. Another reason is that the most mobile joints are found in the extremities.

"It is through the motion of these joints that the pressure is able to move from the trunk to the extremities and back. When there is pressure in a joint, it opens. That joint then has maximal movement and thus is healthy. This is true whether it is a joint in the extremities or one between two vertebrae in the spinal column. Keeping pressure in the body and keeping the joints open is a way of promoting the proper flow of energy and light through our body, and thus insuring our health.

"However, because we've learned very isolated ways of moving, and have repeated them so often, we have to reteach ourselves to be interconnected. We have to pull our light back from the outside world.

"People learn to move certain parts of their bodies disconnected from the others. When you learn to reconnect your body, each movement is made with the whole body. The body begins to act interconnectedly."

He motioned for me to push against his arm which he had raised in front of him. He told me to push as hard as I could. I could not move him.

"You can sustain a blow from the outside with all the pressure in your body," he said, "even though the blow might just be to your arm. Or, you can focus all of this pressure in a motion from the inside out, with a wavelike action that can be like a hammer on a nail." The next thing I knew, I was on the ground again. He motioned for me to get up.

7

"Tension contracts the connective tissue in the sac and prevents energy from flowing through," he continued. "This isolates one part of the body from another. Deep relaxation eases this tension and allows for intercommunication among body systems."

Then he did something I had never seen him do before. He took off his shirt and began to move. He was in a typical martial arts stance. His movements were snakelike, backward and forward, and from side to side.

"Watch closely!" he said. "Pay close attention!" He turned his waist to the right and moved his right arm out. I could see something ripple up his torso and out his arm. He slowly turned his waist to the left, and I saw that same rippling action go out his left arm. He repeated this motion over and over.

"This is how we move pressure. Come and feel!" he said, instructing me to put one hand on his abdomen and another on his shoulder, as he continued moving.

"If you touch me, you won't forget," he said. "We're trying to teach your body, not your chattering mind. Someday when you need the information, this sensory memory will be there to remind you.

"Remember that I told you the body is one big sac. It's like a sac of water being held by gravity," Huang said. "When you want to move that pressure from your torso, which is where the greatest mass of water is, out to your arms, you use a hydraulic system. It's like squeezing a plastic sac of water. You push one place and the pressure moves to the opposite place. Pressure is naturally moved throughout the body by motion, such as walking, turning, and falling." He grinned as I took a step back.

"There is a vertical stretching that goes on in the body," he continued, "and another that twists the body from side to side. You can increase this pressure, and direct it, by the manipulation of your joints. This is only possible because of the interconnectedness of the body.

"When the body is interconnected, we can begin to experience our fluidity. Then, we can learn to pressurize and move this fluidity. Lastly, we can change this pressure into light."

"I don't understand. How can we change this sense of pressure into light?" I asked, at the same time remembering the electrical feel-

8

ing I got every time Huang sent me flying.

"It's something like what takes place at a hydroelectric dam. Water is pressurized and converted into electricity," he replied.

"But that's a big jump. For now, I want you to learn how to reconnect the body and maximize its efficiency of flow."

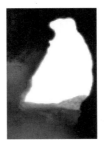

RELAXING

As I was driving home from Huang's house, I began to integrate some of the things he had said. As I relaxed, I could feel how I had increased my sensory possibilities. I was aware of many more things than I was when I was tense.

As I drove, I thought about how in the few years I had been studying with him, Huang had forced me to redefine how I practiced acupuncture and Chinese medicine. Previously, I had worked from mental models and theories. As effective as they sometimes were, I found I was constantly struggling with placing these mental models on the human body. They lacked feeling and texture, and seemed somehow discordant and contradictory. These models and theories only confused me because they lacked a unifying principle.

I looked at the clouds over the mountains and had a realization of how much lighter I had become since studying with Huang. Experiencing my body had become an integral way of understanding and had helped me to qualify many of the different theories I had studied. I now realized that these contradictory theories originally came from the body, and somehow resonated with it.

As I incorporated into my body the concepts Huang had been teaching me—the interconnectedness of gravity, pressure, contact, relaxation, and concentration—I was able to resolve a lot of the contradictions and confusions I had felt. I also started to understand in a tactile way something that I have long believed, that acupuncture and Asian martial arts are an offshoot or remnant of a Chinese yoga. This practice was a way to enlightenment that united the sensory faculties of the body, the uplifting qualities inherent in our emotions, and the psychic and spiritual potentials of our human form.

From Huang I learned that the body offers many possibilities that can be described in many ways. When looked at from the outside, these descriptions may seem contradictory, but when looked at from the inside, they are related like many branches of the same tree.

I remembered something that Huang once told me. He said that I could experience the principles he was teaching me whenever I wanted to, even while I was driving.

The first thing I had to do was just relax. He had told me that relaxation builds pressure. Let it interconnect your body, open your joints, he had said. The key to health and longevity is to keep the joints open.

As I dropped my shoulders and pushed myself down into the seat, creating pressure and opening my joints, I could feel the motion of energy squeeze out from my torso to my extremities and back again.

Huang's use of the word "pressure" had always been difficult for me. I always associated pressure with anxiety, the opposite of relaxation. Now I realized that he was talking about pressure in the sense of oil pressure, like in a car's engine, which had to be at a certain level to allow the car to run properly. If the engine oil pressure is too low, then the engine's "joints," its moving parts, such as the pistons and rods, won't get enough lubrication, and the engine will have problems.

As I continued driving along the winding road, maintaining the pressure in my body, moving the steering wheel from side to side, I put together some pieces of Huang's teachings about body movement. The acupuncture points, I realized, exist at the places where the vertical up and down movements meet the horizontal twisting movements of the body, such as when I turn the steering wheel and my arms go up or down and twist from side to side.

The acupuncture points are where pressure accumulates. This is where we make contact with the world. This is where energy gathers and can be manipulated. I could actually feel how there are places where energy as pressure is increased and directed.

I looked down and saw my wrist and fingers on the steering wheel. Then another realization hit me. Pressure creates space in the joints, allowing for more ways for the joint to move. As I leaned back in the seat and used pressure to open my shoulder joints, I could feel the energy flowing down into my wrist and fingers. My fingers began to tingle. I opened up my elbow and wrist joints. I went on to open my hip, knee, and ankle joints, as well as the spaces in between my spinal column. I directly comprehended through my body that the health of the body is related to the amount of pressure flowing through the spaces between the joints. With more pressure, the moving knowledge that a joint contains can better express its potential.

As I drove further, I remembered how Huang had talked about how the earth was like the body, a body of light. I imagined the earth in the shape of a globe, with its lines of latitude and longitude. Suddenly my body lit up, and I could see that the meridians in my body were like the lines of latitude and longitude on the globe. As I moved back and forth, and side to side, on the winding road, I could feel the pressure in my body pump the energy along the meridian lines.

I could feel the meridians as rivers of pressure and light that flow through the sac of connective tissue. These meridians are the main thoroughfares interconnecting the many regions of the body. I realized that when the joints are moving freely, the acupuncture points and associated meridians are stimulated properly. I focused on the outside of my knee. I felt the pressure ripple out through the rest of my body. I guided it up to my wrist. I felt how my leg and wrist are interconnected. I could then understand that when there is a lack of free motion in the joints it indicates an imbalance in the points, meridians, and associated organs.

As the rush of realizations subsided, I thought about the idea of the connective tissue. I began to think about how Western medical thought has tried to encapsulate acupuncture. Because of the effectiveness of acupuncture, the Western scientific community has been trying to understand how it works. They have postulated that the acupuncture meridians follow nerve pathways, and that the effects of acupuncture are due to the stimulation of the nerves. This theory had always fallen short of describing all of the effects acupuncture can produce, and often the acupuncture meridians don't follow the nerve pathways at all.

I then put together Huang's analogy of the body being a one big sac of luminous pressure, with the Western view of the connective tissue and fascia. Huang was right. Seeing the body as a sac of connective tissue was a way to link some of the Eastern views of the body with modern Western medical thought.

With one model I could think about the theories as well as feel them in my own body. I felt grateful to Huang for what he had taught me.

Still, I wondered how Huang's concepts related to the emotional and spiritual side of my life. I needed to pose this question to another teacher of mine, whom I would be seeing soon.

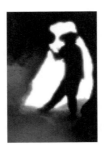

REFLEXIONES:
CRACKING THE PATTERNS

I have been lucky enough in my life to find a teacher—who in this book I call Esmeralda—to show me how to reconnect with the magic of the world, how to break out of the consensual reality of my learned behavior, and how to roam more freely in the magical world that is my birthright.

She taught me that the body is a slide, a transparency, a living metaphor, a holographic representation one chooses through one's belief system to present to the world. She showed me that what I choose to believe about myself determines how I interface with the world, and how that is reflected in what is happening in my life.

Esmeralda was a very exacting person. Her teaching was both concise and precise. The most important thing that I learned from Esmeralda was to be a neutral and clear observer. This teaching has been indispensable. She taught me that my ego, or my learned behavior, wants to perpetuate itself by making me feel either very superior and wonderful or very inferior and a victim. Esmeralda taught me to move through this dichotomy by becoming very neutral and clear with myself. Instead of making me colder towards myself, becoming a neutral and clear observer has allowed me to become more loving and compassionate towards myself and more accepting of others.

Esmeralda taught me that seeing people as superior or inferior was not only something I did within the confines of who I believed myself to be, but that I viewed the world in these terms all the time. She showed me that I would either take an inferior position and expect the world to become my version of superior, or the reverse. She would laugh when she told me that I wasted so much energy maintaining those postures, then always go on to say that neutrality was the only way through it.

I will be forever grateful to her for that, because actualizing this perspective has enabled me to be more accepting of who I am. It has also allowed me to conserve and accumulate energy. This energy has empowered me to move between the cracks of who I perceive myself to be and to become something greater.

Esmeralda taught me to apply this state of neutrality to a strategy of how to relate to the world. She called this strategy "the male-female agreement." Esmeralda showed me that, by using the male-female agreement as a way to examine my life, I would have a very efficient method to track my progress through the quagmire of my learned behavior.

The male-female agreement gave me a sense of direction, something I could lean on in times of stress and confusion. I can now see that, if I had not had this strategy in the midst of the chaos that was created when I began to disassemble my learned behavior, the end result would have been that the patterns of my learned behavior would have reestablished themselves easily. I saw that when we disassemble our learned behavior, we need to have something else available. If I had not had the male-female agreement to support me, the cracks between those patterns, that now have become doors through which I can move into other worlds, would never have opened.

Another of Esmeralda's important teachings is that gathering energy is a way of measuring change or growth. Esmeralda told me that it is important to experience that we're making changes and that something is happening to us, but that in order to have real change, we must create an empty space and maintain it so that it can be filled with energy and spontaneity. Using the male-female agreement to break down my learned behavior was the method I employed to begin to "round up" my potential energy.

Through this process, I've learned to identify myself more as a flow than as a static "me." In an external sense, gathering more energy and seeing myself more as a flow has allowed me to connect with other people and the world in a fuller and more complete way. As a result, I have become much more comfortable about experiencing who I am apart from my conditioned way of thinking.

Through Esmeralda's teachings, I learned that there was something inside of me that was seeking completion with a Bigger Dream and that healing others was about connecting them to this Bigger Dream. Esmeralda emphasized that the male-female agreement is not an end in itself. It is only a method—a strategy—to navigate through our learned behavior and to gather energy. By untangling myself from my learned behavior, I began to experience my true affection for life and saw that this affection, in and of itself, is the great healer.

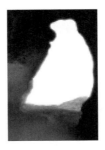

VOLITION:
THE INCANDESCENT PROJECTOR

There is an impulse inside of us that is like a pressure, a light, which is the desire to unite with the world outside, that wants to experience our totality. This can only happen when the luminous membrane that surrounds our body cell and separates our inside from the outside is very sensitive and elastic. It takes a lot of energy to make the pressure from the inside strong enough to keep this membrane stretched out, and allow an unimpeded flow of energy to move between inside and outside.

— Esmeralda

It's magical finding water flowing in the desert. Approaching Esmeralda's house, smelling the water and looking at the cotton woods hanging golden over my head, I realized that Esmeralda's house was an oasis for me. Not only an oasis as life hidden from the heat of the desert sun, but also an oasis for my being, where I could be replenished and recharged.

Birds were singing and rustling in the trees as I neared the doorway. Swallows swooped through the eaves. Esmeralda was standing in the entrance, and I could feel the transformation happening already. Through her powerful yet relaxed presence, I was able to contact what she called the "knowing body," something beyond the way I normally thought of myself. It allowed me the opportunity to feel bigger, more expansive, actively at peace.

Greeting me, she gestured that I follow her into her house. She led me into the living room where I sat down in a white fluffy chair. While I waited for her to make tea, I admired the artistic touches apparent wherever I looked.

I was looking at a bowl of clear water with flowers floating in it when Esmeralda walked in with a teapot and cups. She settled into the chair next to mine, looking at me with a beaming smile.

"Have you changed over yet?"

I smiled and replied that I thought so.

"It's the changing over that allows us to talk in this other way. It lets us talk in pictures," she said.

She offered me some cheese and crackers with my tea, and I declined.

"I hear you've been seeing that old Huang more often these days," she said jokingly.

"He called me the other day, and we had a long talk about you. He told me he'd taught you to see and feel the body as a luminous sac of pressure.

"Well, there's much more to it." She leaned over, poured us each a cup of tea, then sat back with her teacup in her hand.

"Let's play with old Huang's idea," she continued. "It's a good way to look at the body, but it's even better if we look at our whole being as a luminous cell."

She leaned forward, put her teacup down, and leaned back.

"Can you remember when you were womb-bound?"

I put my teacup down and leaned back. Settling in, I got a picture, and then a feeling, of myself in the womb.

I never knew whether it was from the tea, or her, or her house, but when she talked to me, my mind always became very clear, and it was easy to visualize what she was saying. Sometimes the pictures were so clear that I wondered if she was talking to me, or if she was sending sensations and pictures directly from her body to mine.

"Can you sense the luminous cell around you?" she asked. "Your navel is connecting you to that luminosity. You're floating, feeling no need to breathe or eat, just being nurtured by this radiance. This luminous cell is the membrane through which you perceive and through which nourishment is funneled into you.

"Stay there for a moment and feel it with all of your being. Can you remember what happened to that radiance? Can you remember that you still have a luminous cell? The fact is that now you eat and breathe through a bigger luminous sac. You exchanged the amniotic sac, through which you perceived and made contact with the world, for a much larger membrane which became the screen against which all of your perceptions are cast." She leaned forward and looked at me intently.

"There's a luminous bubble around you. I'm knocking on it, and the bubble shivers from my touch," she said, looking at me mischievously.

I felt confused, and it must've shown on my face.

"Don't get linear on me," she said softly. "Keep the multidimensional feeling going."

"Words are very difficult, but they can be like little nuggets of energy, or light, we toss back and forth. In the silent spaces between words, images form. Allow my words to make pictures. Stretch yourself. Stretch your dream fibers. Feel what I am saying." She paused to let this sink in.

"There's a pressure exerted on this membrane from the outside all of the time. Not only the atmospheric pressure that you might think of, but also the pressures of emotions, cultural expectations, psychic influences, my perceptions, and everything else that the world constantly throws at you. One of the reasons that you feel different when you're here is because of the peculiar nature of the pressure I exert."

I was amazed at how I could play with these holographic images, images that were not just visual, but that could be felt, touched, smelled, and listened to as she summoned them up.

"Let's put a little twist in this," she continued, "and bring it together with some of the things Huang was talking about. Think of the body as if it were a three-dimensional slide. At its very core, going up and down the trunk, there is a light that shines the body's pattern out onto that membrane or screen that we just talked about. It's like a long thin light that extends from your perineum to the crown of your head. It radiates light in all directions through the slide of your physical body, which is what Huang called your sac. This image is projected onto an outer luminous membrane which is created by the combined inputs of all of our senses."

As I sat there, I could feel how all of my senses created a luminous membrane around me.

"It's different from the kind of projector you might be thinking of, because it's not just projecting visual images, but also tactile, olfactory, and auditory images, every kind of sensory stimulus you can feel!" she continued.

"Think of a flow of vibrational energy moving back and forth. We take it in through our senses in various ways, and we split it up into a spectrum, tasting, hearing, seeing, and so forth. Think of that vibrational flow as being one thing that can be translated through the combination of senses of our choice. We can hear a movement, or taste a smell, or see a sound!

"The light becomes outward flowing energy by shining through your body. It goes out and contacts the membrane, making it luminous, creating a place where impressions are made. Upon contact, multisensual people, animals, trees, water, fire are perceived, as the impressions are interpreted."

The cadence of Esmeralda's voice changed.

"If you can change the slide, or your physical body," she said slowly, leaning over and touching my knee, "then what you see on your screen changes. The physical body stores your perceptual patterns. Once your idea of your body and who you think you are changes, your reality also changes.

"Remember when you were here last time, and we put a candle in that tin lamp shade with designs cut into it, and enjoyed the shadows it cast on the wall? That's another way to visualize the slide and its projection on the outer membrane.

"Let's go back to Huang's idea of pressure, and integrate it into the images and feelings you are experiencing here," she continued.

"The light in the projector is a pressure that flows out through the slide of the physical body and stretches this outer membrane against the pressure and light from the outside, like blowing up a balloon. This creates the luminous cell that we are.

"When we have a very resilient membrane it allows for a great variety of contact and interaction between our side of the membrane and the world. In this way, we can maximize our feeling of wholeness and health."

A question arose inside of me. Esmeralda's pictures in my mind began to lose their clarity and were replaced with some images of my own. I was seeing people as luminous cells of energy, some of them collapsing and wrinkled, others strong and vibrant. I noticed the physical bodies of the ones that were collapsing and wrinkled. As I watched, they got weaker, and the outer membrane folded up around them. I realized that some of them were similar to patients that I saw in my clinic.

I asked whether these luminous cells can wrinkle up and get hard and brittle.

"Ah, you anticipate me!" she said. "This is exactly what happens.

"Let me use a few words to help you fill in these pictures. I'm sure Huang told you about how when we're young, we have lots of pressure. As we grow older, our learned repetitive patterns cause our inner pressure and resilience to diminish. Our outer membrane starts to stiffen and begins to collapse in on itself under the influence of the pressure coming in from the outside. This creates a wrinkling effect. The kinds of wrinkles are determined by the configuration of pressure we maintain on the inside of our luminous membrane. When the pressure inside can no longer withstand the pressure from the outside, the membrane ruptures."

"What happens then?" I asked.

"Death."

"Is there any way to keep the membranes from wrinkling and collapsing?" I asked.

"Yes, and that's what this teaching is really all about," she said. "The answers to that question will come to you only when you incorporate the teaching into your body. You have to understand that incorporating these concepts takes a long time. You must begin to feel them at a living level.

"I'm not teaching you these ideas for you to grab with your mind, get a little rush, and then go on to the next thing. I'm teaching you how to redirect your whole life."

She stopped for a minute. "A lot of inertia is built up through your life experiences and works inside of you at a level which you can't even imagine. To go against this is really hard work. Slow, hard work.

"What I want to do is to take this knowledge that I am summoning up within you, allow you to feel it, and then teach you how to integrate it into your body so that you can remember it. This is the only way real change can be sustained.

"In fact, enough of this sitting around! It's important to get body motion into teaching." She laughed.

We got up and stretched.

"Stand up and face that wall," Esmeralda said, pointing to the wall on our right.

I walked over and put my nose up against the wall.

"Notice that your ears actually face the wall, and that your eyes look at the wall," she said. "See that your nose points towards the wall, and that your mouth points towards the wall, too! Even the navel area, where we receive nourishment, faces the wall. All of this is in the front of your body.

"Now step back," she said.

I did.

"Now spread your arms wide open," she said. "Now close them in front of you. Do you see how they function most effectively with the part of you that faces the wall, rather than behind your back? Look at your feet. They are facing the wall too! Most of the interacting that we do as people has to do with the front part of our bodies.

"Notice your genitals! Where are they facing? The wall, right?"

Suddenly I felt an arm at my neck and found myself falling down onto the floor. She stood over me.

"Stay down there!" she commanded. "The back part is our Yang or defensive part." To my surprise, she began kicking me! I

24

pulled into a fetal position to protect myself.

"You respond so well!" she laughed. "That position is a very protected one. Notice that all of those parts we were talking about before, your eyes, nose, face, ears, mouth, chest, abdomen, and genitals, are now all shielded by your Yang or defensive part, from the back part of your head to your heels."

"Now open up and lie on your back."

"Are you kidding? I'm afraid you might kick me!" I said.

"Aha!" she said. "Exactly! You got it! You now know which part of your body is soft and vulnerable. It is from this soft and vulnerable part of your body that you primarily interact with the world."

She motioned for me to stand up.

"So you can see that our protective part is in the back. It's through the front that we interact with the world. It is in the front where we use our hands to put food in our mouths. It's toward the front that we usually walk. Furthermore, it is by means of the faculties in our front that we interact with each other."

"Face the wall again," she said. I nervously followed her order. The next thing I felt was her back against mine.

"You can feel my back against yours, can't you?" she asked.

Not waiting for me to respond, she read me the verses that were written on a framed piece of parchment hung on the wall across the way:

> The wind
> swirls about,
> shrieking as it passes.

> Leaving all
> stretched to form
> for it to flow.

She stopped.
"How do you feel?" she asked.
"Fine!"

"You don't feel uncomfortable, do you?"

"No," I said.

"We are going to try something now," she said. "I want you to turn around slowly."

Maintaining contact, we began to turn slowly at the same time. As I turned, I felt uncomfortable, even panicked because of our closeness. As we continued turning, I was overwhelmed by the stimulus. The next thing I knew, we were nose to nose and eye to eye and belly to belly. I felt Esmeralda's breasts pressed against my chest, her abdomen pressed against mine. While she seemed totally relaxed, I found I had to drop my eyes to reduce the intensity. We stood like this for a long moment.

"Does this feel comfortable?" she asked.

"No!" I said.

"This is what I am going to teach you. How to be this close to a person, and be internally silent, and still feel relaxed.

"What makes you uncomfortable are all those things you learned when you were young," she said smiling. "When you try to be still in close proximity to another person, what will arise is all of the fear and paranoia that went into making your idea of your body.

"Over the course of your life, you have given away much energy, much pressure, so that you are not at peace with yourself. You have been taught incorrectly that you can find peace in yourself by trading energy with other people.

"You have to learn how to maintain pressure within yourself from your own resources, even while relating to other people. I can stand next to you, and I can feel peaceful and strong. But for you it is hard. You have lost much energy to your repetitive patterns. The ways that you connect with yourself and to the world are no longer efficient or resilient. They are worn out. You must learn to make those sensations that reach out strong, resilient, and pliable.

"Now let's get back to the idea of the luminous cell," she said, returning to her chair and sitting down.

I walked back.

"What does looking at the wall and seeing that most of my sense organs are in front of me, and getting kicked around to show me how to protect myself, have to do with the luminous cell?" I asked.

"That was a mouthful." She laughed. "We are thinking the same thing. We are working very closely now. Our bodies are really talking." She winked. "Our luminous cells are in some ways joined!"

I sat down in my chair, and she continued.

"The luminous cell is an egg-like structure that we live in. Our back is up against the shell of this egg, in the same way that your body is pressing against the chair that you're sitting in. Feel how the majority of the egg is in front of you."

Esmeralda looked at me. She must've felt how tired I was.

"I want you to remember this for when we meet again," she said. "You're full now, it's time for you to digest this."

The next day I left her house feeling very different, somehow bigger and more expanded.

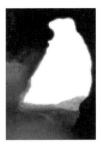

LUMINOUS CELLS

A few days later I was in a restaurant, eating a bowl of good spaghetti. For some reason when I eat, the energy in my body descends, I begin to relax, and my mind goes slower. As I relaxed, I began experiencing a feeling similar to what I had felt with Esmeralda. As this feeling filled me, I saw the world differently. It was as if I could touch things with my eyes. It was as if I was in a gelatinous world, made of clear, vibrating jello. Everything was iridescent, glowing and refracting like light inside of a jellyfish.

I was reminded of an old Hopi legend that says that Spider Woman used her spittle to make life. The whole world was made of a spittle-like substance similar to the white of an egg, fluid yet full of life.

I noticed the people around me. Most of them were in pairs or small groups, facing one another. I could feel/see their interaction. Through their conversation and movement, their bodies were communicating with one another.

Each person had his or her own individual luminous cell, and when they came together their luminous cells would merge. The pair or group would then communicate within these bubbles. I saw how the concentration of sensory inputs was in the front of each person's cell, allowing them to lock into each other.

The tables were packed very tightly in the restaurant, and wherever people were interacting, their attention was glued together. The concentration required to maintain this communication insulated them from what was going on around them. I realized how their luminosity and attention were the same thing.

I dug my fingernails into my hand a few times to make sure I wasn't just seeing things. This gesture made me laugh at myself, but the experience didn't go away.

As I watched the people in the restaurant, I noticed that many of the interactions were similar. The women that were together seemed to be making certain agreements, and these agreements had a texture, a feeling, a light that accompanied them. The agreements of the men who were locked in communication had a different tonal resonance. I saw that a man and a woman together had still another feeling or glow. Each of these types were different from each other yet somehow related.

After lunch, I left the restaurant and walked around. While walking I began to feel how I was a luminous cell, too. My senses were connected to the edges of my cell with fibers of light. It was exhilarating to feel this connection.

I walked down to the Plaza. The light breeze was like a fluid current moving around the branches and leaves, somehow nurturing the living things it caressed.

I began playing with the luminosity I felt around me. I moved in close to a man selling *carnitas*—meat-filled tortillas—on the corner. I could feel when our luminous cells began to merge, and our bodies began to communicate. He didn't react, but I knew he felt me as I felt him, like when someone in a passing car is staring at you, or when you know someone with sunglasses is looking at you even though you can't see their eyes.

I moved on and began experimenting to see how close I could get to other people before I felt them with my luminous cell. I related with person after person in this way. I started calling the feeling of making contact with them "brushing my fibers."

I then understood that one of the reasons I liked to interact with people was to have my fibers brushed. I realized that uniting momentarily with others, and their slightly different perceptions of the world, opened me up to new combinations of experience. This gave me a feeling of revitalization as my set ways of contacting the world were brushed loose.

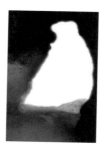

THE BODY KNOWS

The first snow had fallen. At last I could rest. The earth seemed to be giving me permission to go inside. There were many activities I knew I didn't have to do now, not because they weren't there to do, but because I felt like the time for doing them was over. The air was brisk and refreshing, invigorating yet relaxing. There was a sense of completion in it. The seeds were snuggling into the ground, just beginning to feel where they were. The still pressure of the falling snow made me feel like I was also a seed settling down into the earth as I descended the steps into Huang's studio.

I could see the *bagua*, the eight trigrams of the *I Ching*, arranged in a circle in the brick on the studio floor, with the yin yang symbol in its center. Huang was standing by the window, sipping a hot cup of tea, watching the snow dance in the courtyard. He turned around and acknowledged me with a small bow and a huge smile.

"I'm glad to see that you came back," he said.

He always had a way of throwing me off balance, if not with a shove across the room then with his words. Since I came to him for weekly lessons, it made me nervous when he said incongruous things like that.

It wasn't that I didn't like him. I loved the feeling of being around him. It was a strange contradiction. On the one hand, when

33

in his presence, my body felt energized and alive in a very special way. On the other hand, I always had the feeling around him that something new was about to come out of me, something I was afraid I couldn't handle.

Huang put his teacup down and waved me over. He got into the stance for a two-man martial exercise, and indicated for me to join him. We began shifting our weight back and forth from one foot to the other, engaging each other wrist to wrist, practicing what he called "sticking." This was an exercise which involved engaging another person as sensitively as possible, merging with their energy, and in this way understanding their movement and intention.

"Too hard! Soft on the outside, hard on the inside. Steel wrapped with cotton!" he said, stopping the motion.

"Let's try something to soften you up. Let's go back to the same exercise. This time I want you to be very, very sensitive. You lead. Move your hands any way you want. Move back and forth in your stance. I'll follow you with my body, maintaining contact with my arms against yours."

We started to move. I moved my arms, shifted my weight from my front leg to my back leg. Huang seemed to be with me wherever I was. I tried being tricky. I tried to figure out ways to lose him. It had no effect, and finally I relaxed into moving the way I felt like moving.

There came a point when I didn't know if Huang was moving first, or I was. It seemed as though our luminous cells had merged. The more I relaxed, the more I could feel the knowledge he had in his body flow into mine. His movement was a new language. This is what I had come to him to learn.

As that realization surfaced in my mind, he bumped me with his hand and admonished me to pay attention.

"Put your realizations into motion!" he said. "Realize and stay fluid. Integrate the realization into your body as you are realizing it."

I couldn't quite incorporate what he was saying. To me, realizing was a thinking process that took me out of my body and into my head. To Huang, realizing was a bodily process. Once again I felt stupid, as I often did around him.

I had once told him about this, about how stupid I felt. He said

34

that it takes a long time for the body to relearn what it already knows, and that the times that I felt stupid were often the times when I was learning the most.

My mind drifted for a moment, and I remembered a time when I was with him and felt like I knew what I was doing. Then the feeling of stupidity arose, as it always seemed to, and I suddenly felt I knew nothing. He had corrected my posture. I began to defend my actions, giving excuses for my supposed awkwardness. When I did that, he signaled for me to stop talking and said, "Just relax, feel stupid. Let your body talk."

Remembering this relaxed me, and I felt myself in the room again. The thoughts dissolved back into my body. I became the movement.

My body was unable to sustain the charge of our combined energies for very long. This new language he was teaching me required an unbelievable amount of energy. My legs began to tire. Finally, when I thought my legs were about to explode, he stopped and motioned me over to the window where the snow was still falling.

"It takes a lot of energy to regain the fluid elasticity that you had when you were young," Huang said. "When you were young, you were very aware of how bodies talked to other bodies. To remember and relearn how to do that requires a lot of concentration and practice, far beyond anything you can imagine.

"To even realize that you have these capabilities, you have to allow this new energy, or light, to flow in your body. Then you have to work on it, practicing diligently to stabilize it, to allow this energy to become functional."

I nodded, acknowledging that I was just beginning to see how far I had to go.

"Don't worry," he said, "it's just that you're not operating with a full deck right now." He chuckled.

After a few minutes, we began a new exercise. He used the same principles, but this time the exercise was free form, moving around the room. From the outside, the repetition of this exercise would have been very tedious to watch. From the inside, however, nuggets of awareness were being shifted and shared.

Then it happened, the feeling of stupidity set in again. All of a sudden the motions I was making didn't seem creative. They seemed repetitive and dead. I became self-conscious. I worried that I was boring Huang.

My uncertainty didn't seem to bother him. He maintained contact no matter how self-conscious I felt. He kept pressuring me, even though he was barely touching me. Finally I felt so stupid I gave up. I stopped trying and relaxed. Then something else took over. I didn't know if he was following me or if I was following him. Once again knowledge flowed.

It seemed as though I could only take so much of this. Even with Huang around lending me energy through inspiration, direction, and his physical presence, I could only maintain this state of concentration for a short period of time. It was like building up a new muscle. Soon this fluid, flexible way of moving wore me down, because I didn't have the energy to maintain this pressure.

I finally had to break off. I shook out my legs and loosened up my arms as I moved toward the cool air by the windows. This was one of those occasions when I hoped Huang would tell me one of his stories that seemed to live in another time and space. The descriptions he painted in these stories seemed to transport me to another dimension. But, instead of telling a story, he went up the stairs to get some fresh tea.

I looked out into the whirling snow, motion still pulsing through my veins. A memory began to seep into my consciousness, coming from all parts of my body at once. Thirteen again, in front of a window. Moving from foot to foot, feeling nauseous, suffocating in the gas-heated gym. Junior high school dance about to begin. Lining up, girls on one side, us on the other, separated by the teachers, the referees. Looking down at my feet as the music began, terrified that if I raised my eyes and looked over, the confusion would smash me.

How was I going to move with someone over there?

Finally dancing, moving awkwardly, sticks and stubs for arms and legs. Feeling drained when it was over, wishing I could be outside, running in the rain.

I found myself back in Huang's studio, realizing I had never

36

recovered from that early teenage experience. Huang was looking at me, studying me intently.

"Where were you?" he asked.

I told him about the dance, my awkwardness. It was as if I remembered something I had either blocked out or not wanted to feel.

He put his teacup down.

"That's great!" he said. "You have gathered enough energy to remember that! You have created enough pressure inside your luminous cell to go back to that time.

"When we are younger, we naturally have more pressure. We're really whirlwinds of energy, full of life and potential. What happens to most of us as we get older is that we lose pressure, and can't access or remember things in the past."

I stopped him.

"I can't believe that you were this way too!" I said. "You're just trying to make me feel better."

"No, it's true," he said. "And, because I was once like you, I can understand the formidable foes that you now face.

"Don't deceive yourself, they are formidable! The task before you is to reclaim your true inheritance, to understand what you really are."

He paused, then continued emphatically.

"When you work on rebuilding pressure from within, you can teach yourself to remember experiences with your whole body. This is a different kind of remembering, a more total remembering. It's not just the flat linear remembering that occurs when you're watching reruns of your own personal drama, but actually remembering with your whole being."

I felt a little baffled by what he had just told me.

"Say that again?" I asked.

Huang began to speak in a very dry, factual tone that I rarely heard from him.

"Throughout the whole body cell we store memories in patterns of connective tissue. As we create more pressure and expand from the inside, we are able to contact ways of perceiving that we had in the past, but were buried.

37

"When we get older, we lose pressure through constant repetition of patterns, and our view of the world narrows. So we have to rekindle the spirit within us and give it a home. We have to recall the light that we are expending on a limited view of the world and redirect it. This creates a pressure.

"Through cultivation," he said, "this pressure can be made to relight our being. Old rooms inside of ourselves that have long been abandoned come back to life. Our dismembered bodies come back together.

"We have the energy to access ways of putting together the world that we had lost. And we have the energy to re-member," he said, jokingly.

"We can only remember a place when we're in it," he added.

I was really confused now.

"Do you mean like when I drive by a town I used to live in, and a lot of these thoughts and memories of when I lived there rush back? Or like, if I went back to that gym, and looked out of that same window, and remembered what had happened there?"

"That's not exactly what I'm talking about," Huang replied.

"We are talking about two different things. What you felt here was a result of gaining pressure from the inside through movement and concentration, and the boost from my energy. Remember that: Inside!

"What you asked me about has to do with pressure from the outside. Remember that: Outside! Pressure from the outside can produce a remembrance. This happens to everybody. For example, when you come into my studio, other things that have happened to you here float to the surface. This is very helpful because it gives you a series of memories upon which to build. It's important to remember, however, that it is only a backdrop to the real work inside. It is only through creating pressure from the inside that we can sustain and integrate knowledge."

"How would this apply to people I know that like to go to certain places they call power spots?" I asked. "They report that they feel somehow transformed by the experience."

"You can go to certain places on the earth, and get energy there.

38

But without direction and pressure from the inside, you have no way of storing the energy you momentarily feel. When you leave, whatever energy you may have gained soon dissipates, because you can't remember or access it in the totality with which you experienced it. You may remember that you had a nice time, but you won't have the energy to access the memory through your body.

"One thing that happens by building pressure from the inside is that you fill up your reservoir of energy," he said. "When you increase this pool of energy on the inside, or increase the pressure, then you begin to have real control. You create a vessel within which you can store your light.

"You didn't have to go to the junior high gym to have your memory. You can gain enough pressure to remember the way your body felt inside, instead of having to travel around physically, which isn't very efficient." He paused.

"Also, as you begin to gain more and more pressure, you no longer demand the same tedious repetition of outside stimuli to maintain your idea of who you are. So you're easier to be around."

He stopped and chuckled, seemingly at himself.

"I grew up in a culture of secrets," he said. "The Chinese, for various reasons, have developed secrecy to a high art. These reasons were for the most part selfish: to preserve money, power, and prestige. But there are unselfish reasons for keeping secrets.

"Sometimes the internal flow of knowledge can also be seen as secretive. However, here a principle is only a secret if you don't have the capacity, the persistence, or the strength to understand it. So, I'm not dealing with secrets, even though to you it may sometimes seem so. What I do is impart knowledge in terms of appropriateness." He chuckled again.

I then had to ask him, "Well, what were you chuckling about now?"

"I was thinking about telling you a real secret," he said. "I remembered how little I really understood it when I first heard it. A real secret that I had to work my ass off to understand."

"Why should something be hard to understand if it's explained well?" I asked.

39

"Some things are learned very slowly. It's one thing to hear the words, and it's another to allow them to grow inside of you.

"Now listen closely, and we'll see how you do. I'll be telling you this over and over again in many different ways. In fact, I have been telling it to you ever since you first started studying with me.

"It was a secret that's now about to come out." He laughed. "You know, sometimes, the jokes we have with ourselves are the funniest."

He suddenly became serious.

"The real secret is getting the volition to flow through the connective tissue," he said. "The question is," he continued, "how do you get your volition to flow through the movements of your body, not only within yourself, but within your interactions with other people?"

I reacted with puzzled expression.

He looked at me and said, "After all, we are the way that we relate.

"Volition is really the most concentrated of pressures," Huang explained. "Let's call it seed pressure. It is our luminous essence. Volition grows as it moves throughout our connective tissue. The luminous cell is the container for our being. Your body is where you stabilize and sustain the power of volition. It is the platform from which you can learn to fly.

"Your work here is to loosen up your body so that your luminous essence can flow freely."

He motioned for me to join him. We stood facing each other, touching wrists.

"One last thing," he said. He touched me with what felt like an electric charge and I went reeling across the room.

Again, I had that time-warp feeling you have when you're in an accident. I always wondered how he did that. Huang often told me he was trying to teach me to do that but, for the life of me, I didn't know where inside me it was going to come from.

"In a martial way, this is how we use that principle," he said.

He then walked over to me, chuckling.

"I'm going to tell you another secret. Listen carefully," he said, pausing for a moment.

"The body is not what you think it is, but it becomes what you think it is."

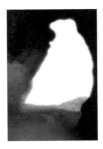

Pressure from Within

I t was getting cold again, up in the high desert. I usually liked to
go south this time of year, to see the migrating birds and soak in
some hot springs. This time I had a special reason to go south.
Huang had recommended that I meet a friend of his, a healer named
Eulogio Rodriguez who lived on the Mexican border.

I shuffled around town for awhile getting ready. I packed my
truck and drove off around mid-morning.

As I moved further away from town, I began to disconnect from
my life there. I could feel my memories and associations lifting. It
was a relief to get into the silence of the open desert.

I had found that when I drove for long distances, it was like a
meditation. A book I once read said that cars were like caves. I chuckled to myself, thinking that this was especially true when you made
your car into a nest of papers and old clothes like some people I knew.

I thought about Huang, and how serious he always seemed to
be. Then I remembered Esmeralda telling me that that was just the
way that he was sometimes, that I should see him when they got together. Perhaps sometime I would.

I continued driving. Finally, after getting about twenty miles
out of town, I felt I had really left. I was in the clear mind of the desert
once again.

As I drove, I practiced some of the exercises Huang had shown me. He told me that these were good to do when I was driving, or in the mall, or standing in line at the bank. As I did them now, I felt my butt pressing hard into the seat. I wondered how the seat held up.

I created more pressure, and suddenly cringed, wondering if a spring was going to come flying out. That would be something to tell old Huang!

Finally I reached the crest of a hill. The panoramic view of desert, mountain, and sky opened up before me. I began thinking about a friend of mine who was a psychic. She made predictions for other people. People called her from all over the United States to find answers for their problems, or to get some kind of inspiration to help them feel okay about who they were, or thought they were.

I realized that most of their problems were just variations on their repetitive patterns. They would ask about their next love affair, their job, when to invest money. In short, they asked how to better entrench themselves in the same patterns that were driving them to seek help in the first place. Little did they know that this repetitive choreography was only digging them in deeper.

Knowing this person, and feeling what it was like to be around her, it seemed as though this psychism hadn't really helped her life. It might have given her more ability to understand the patterns around her and around other people; however, since her focus was based on the manipulation of these patterns, it was still based on the patterns, and not on breaking them down to nurture a new awareness.

In fact, Huang had said, when I asked him about psychics, that there was a danger there. He said that a person could be so dazzled by the power of manipulation and prognostication, that they would get even more stuck in their patterns than those who hadn't developed any psychic ability at all.

He also said that, without the pressure coming from the inside, no manipulation of the external pressures was really going to make much difference in terms of a being's ability to experience living. It was similar to what Huang told me about people who went to power places to gather energy. My acquaintance would move in these psychic worlds, which had more energy, but she was unable to stabilize that light in her body or her life.

As I kept driving, watching the mountains flow by, my thoughts drifted and reformed.

I thought about an acupuncture teacher I once had who always asked would-be students why they wanted to study with him. If they replied that it was because they wanted to help people, he would turn them away. He would only allow them to study with him if they chose to use the study of medicine primarily as a method of self-discovery.

He knew that truly helping people was a natural by-product of self-discovery. Going within was the key to regenerating oneself, and this constant regeneration was the way to touch the pulse of life, for oneself and for others.

Thinking about my old teacher, I saw that there was a progression to my own regeneration. At first I thought that healing was fixing someone who was hurt. If they couldn't function properly within their normal context, I felt compelled to try and patch them up. In many instances I was successful, but as I continued to practice, it was less and less fulfilling to assist people in this way. I felt forced to change.

Looking back, I realized that I was gaining pressure, and as a result, found that there was more to healing than just pasting people together and putting them back on the street.

When I looked more closely at what I was doing, I discovered that the way I attempted to assist people was a direct reflection of the way that I wanted to be helped myself. There was a greater healing to be sought inside myself than simply becoming more effective within my socially conditioned roles. This then led me to wonder if I would ever know what a true cure really was.

As I drove, I began to look even more deeply within myself, considering my motives for existing. Filled with self-doubt, I knew I needed to find other motives for existing than those conventionally held.

I shivered, and suddenly I became self-involved. My energy plummeted. I felt totally drained and empty. I didn't know who I was. I became afraid. I felt so lonely. I could no longer recognize myself. I felt as if I was dropping into a deep dark hole with no way out. At the same time, I knew I had to find myself.

I had to see Esmeralda. And, although it was out of my way, I had to see her before I continued on my trip to meet Eulogio.

Esmeralda always seemed to know how to push me beyond myself to find myself again.

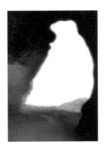

FALLING APART

By the time I pulled up in front of Esmeralda's house, I felt heavy. I didn't feel connected with myself or the world around me. My vibrant sense of aloneness had changed to a real sense of loneliness.

Esmeralda was waiting at my regular parking spot. She opened the car door for me.

"I don't feel so good," I said.

"I can see that," she said. "Come up, we'll have a cup of tea." She looked at me again, rested her chin on her hand for a moment.

"On second thought, let's go for a walk," she said. "Sometimes when we get stuck like this, movement is the best thing. And there's nothing like moving in nature, where everything is in its perfect place, to remind us of our own perfection."

As we walked, Esmeralda encouraged me to talk. I told her about how lonely I felt. She said that these episodes will happen. One of the consequences of building pressure and gathering light in one's body is that one breaks further and further away from the learned behavior of the time.

"When for some reason we can't sustain the pressure we've been cultivating," she continued, "and we are forced to revert to our old way of relating, it is no longer satisfying. That is when the sense of loneliness sets in, because we don't recognize ourselves anymore."

As I walked beside Esmeralda, I started to understand what had happened to me. I had become self-involved in an old way, and my energy had plummeted.

"As we gather more pressure and learn to live differently," Esmeralda continued, "we learn to line ourselves up more properly with gravity in order to sustain our pressure. We learn to be better aligned with heaven and earth, like a plant, or a wild animal."

She paused and looked at me.

"As humans, we have a natural affection in us for our own kind. We have to learn to relate to other humans, because that's part of what being human is. When we make a change and realign ourselves, we need to spread it throughout our range of being human. This stabilizes the change throughout our luminous cell."

Esmeralda continued walking, and was silent for a moment. I listened to the soft sound of our footsteps.

"When we are young, we trade in our natural sense of being between heaven and earth, or a vertical way of maintaining ourselves, for ways of interacting with our family, or horizontal interactions. The family, or our early relations, take our natural sense of affection and twists it. This contorted view of relating creates an unnatural energy bartering system to which we are forced to acquiesce."

We momentarily stopped to admire cottonwood leaves drifting in the creek next to where we were walking. I noticed how the leaves floated on the surface without sinking. The soft mud felt alive under my moccasined feet.

Esmeralda looked at me.

"You come from the womb," she said, "where you are a luminous cell connected to everything, and nurturing flows to you from all sides. After you are born you want to continue receiving this nourishment, but only certain channels are offered to you.

"You trade in the natural homeostasis you had before birth for the pressure you can get from other people. You begin to incorporate the ways of your family. They teach you what they have been taught will make a person best function in society, to the exclusion of all else that you might possibly be.

"Usually," she said, "I would want to shift you quickly out of this place where you are so that you would change to a place that's more receptive to my teaching. However, today I want to just be with you and let you work it out slowly. This will let you see as many of the little steps as possible. These are the little steps you typically go through to get your pressure back. Variations of this loneliness will be with you for a long time yet. You need to learn how to deal with it."

Esmeralda was silent as she led me down to a pool in the canyon. Red rocks were all around us. There was an emptiness in the sky, as if it was waiting for the sunset. We sat in the shade that the rocks cast on the canyon wall.

I felt strange. I could not connect with the beauty around me. It was frustrating. Esmeralda told me to let my body unwind, that she would be my witness. She told me to let myself just be how I was, reaffirm my confidence in myself, and allow my volition to open me up in a natural way.

Esmeralda let me know that whatever I was feeling was acceptable. The sense of judgment I placed on my own feelings fell away, and I began to relax. I also sensed that she was there to help give me direction.

After a while, Esmeralda's voice broke through my thoughts.

"Now that you've felt that it's all right to feel your loneliness with me, let's walk a little more," she said. "Don't leave your loneliness behind, bring it with you. We want to let your loneliness go slowly, so that you can carefully examine the process that you go through."

She rose and we ascended a narrow trail to the top of the canyon. The panoramic view was stupendous. The afternoon light was just turning. Magic was beginning to appear in the air. The winter sun seemed friendly, warming me softly. The snow-covered mountaintops were silhouetted against the crystalline blue sky.

"I hope you brought that feeling with you, and didn't leave it behind," she reminded me.

"Watch!" She stepped onto a large flat rock and began stamping her feet rapidly in tiny solid steps, turning in semicircles, facing the mountain-carved horizon. Her arms hung loosely at her sides. She motioned for me to join her. It took me a while to get the footwork down, especially since I was still feeling heavy. At first it seemed very tiring.

"Watch the horizon with your eyes," she said. "Don't focus on anything. Keep your eyes open as you slowly turn from side to side. Feel the earth. Let yourself feel humble in this vast open space."

As I continued to move, I began to melt into my loneliness. I felt that I was praying rather than dancing, connecting earth and sky through the core of my being. I felt simple and alone. It was fine. More than fine, it was beautiful and complete.

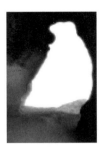

ACTIVATING VOLITION

W e were walking back toward her house. On the way, we stopped at an outcropping of rocks dominated by a pine tree rising from a crevice. The tenacity of the tree's will to live seemed to overpower and pervade this special place. The sun was just beginning to set, and colors filled the sky. The crows were finishing their evening flight.

"Now I am going to indulge you," Esmeralda told me. "Men always seem to need such explanations. They don't seem to make progress without them." She motioned for me to sit against a rock that had been warmed by the sun. I leaned back and she sat down to my left against another rock.

"Volition rises like a spark inside of one's body," she said. "Pressure helps distribute it throughout. Volition is like that internal projector we talked about before. The light from this core illuminates our being. It's like the heart of this pine tree, rising straight up the middle of the trunk, providing sustenance for the tree's unfolding," she said looking over at the pine tree.

"The core wants to interact freely with the outside through our body. It flows out through our beliefs about who we are. These beliefs actually have a structure: The idea we have of our body.

"Our potential as humans is not expressed very well through

our societal training. We need to reactivate our volition to try to re-connect ourselves with our humbleness and the outside. Initially, this energy is distributed through our bodies in the patterns of our old fixations because we don't know any other way. However, as we in-crease our contact with volition, the pressure and then the light from the inside grows. It's more pressure than our old patterns are used to.

"Every time the pressure inside of us builds, our idea of who we are expands a little bit. This process creates what to each of us feels like a falling apart and coming back together, in a wavelike action. The more we relax into this process of volition moving through the body, the faster these waves will become, until we can bring the surge of volition into our life and stabilize it.

"The techniques that Huang is teaching you allow for a smoother flow of volition through your body. This enables your being to go through this process with less wear and tear. If one doesn't have a way of distributing the huge surges of energy through one's body and stabilizing them, diseases can develop.

"In the East, this was called Zen sickness, or meditation sick-ness. These so-called Zen sicknesses could not be treated by an ordi-nary doctor. They were caused by a liberation of light from within that was not able to express itself harmoniously through the body.

"These illnesses are different from ordinary illnesses caused by repetitive ways of moving in the world. The latter are caused by the erosion of our learned behavior by pressure from the outside, whereas the former have to do with an explosion of energy from the inside which is too much for the learned behavior, or one's conditioned idea of the body, to handle.

"Huang in his way, and me in mine, are trying to teach you to unite with your volition. What Huang taught you is so important be-cause without some kind of discipline, or some idea of how to inte-grate this new energy into your body, you might well go crazy," she said.

"If you are working to free yourself from the inside, you will experience an ebb and flow in your body, as volition or your connec-tion with the spirit increases. Each time you fall apart, you experience your humbleness. When you pull yourself together, your self-image

52

will be a little different. This process will be repeated over and over.

"Getting used to the process of falling apart and pulling yourself back together is very important. The trick is, how do you let yourself fall apart without going mad? Better yet, how do you allow who you think you are to come together and fall apart while maintaining contact with the spirit. Once the process is initiated, one needs to learn to flow with it, and great efforts have to be made not to do unnecessary damage to the body.

"In the end," she continued, "the falling apart and coming together don't matter. The ability to maintain contact with the spirit does. That is the point. That is the muscle you're trying to build. You can't really change who you are, or who you think you are, but you can learn to become something greater, and not identify with who you think you are or aren't."

Esmeralda looked over at me.

"You can see that trying to change who you think you are is really a foolish thing. You're trying to get beyond who you think you are."

Esmeralda leaned forward and drew in the soft earth: a figure eight lying on its side. She followed the outline with her finger several times.

While she spoke, she continued moving her finger through the figure eight in the earth. "Our comings and goings, or who we think we are and aren't, are linked together like this. One depends upon the other for its existence. If you move strongly into one, you're driven back into the other one. If you try to work either for or against who you think you are—what is normally referred to as 'changing' yourself—you really never do change! You just stay on the same continuum."

She sat upright, and continued.

"In many cases, people are drawn to drug experiences to experience their spirit. Drugs and alcohol, however, when used repetitively, severely tax the body. Certain religions are based on the same premise. The doomsday preacher will make his parishioners acutely aware of how they are alive in this very moment, because doomsday is about to happen. The preacher and the parishioners are filled with volition, but they have no appropriate way of expressing it through their greatest treasure, their bodies. When they go out into the world of relating, they don't know how to embody their volition and end up contorted."

She stood up, stretched, and began staring down at me, turning her head from side to side. Then she blurted out, "Eat!" I was startled at first.

She began cackling, and then I laughed with her.

"You're hungry, I see," she said. "Let's go!"

When we got back to the house, she said she had the perfect thing for me. A pot of beans and chili that she had cooked yesterday.

"They are always better on the second day," she said. "Maybe they have a little more volition in them. Or is it pressure?" She laughed again. I asked myself why it was that I always had to be around these people who told themselves jokes all the time.

She then asked me if I knew why farts smelled. I said I didn't have the slightest idea, inwardly dreading what was to come.

"So that deaf people can enjoy them too!" she said, and began another round of laughter.

When she had finished laughing, Esmeralda described to me how laughing created a roller coaster of images, that one thing led to another. Yes, she was laughing at the look on my face, but she was laughing at the fact that she was a terrible joke teller, and she was laughing remembering the fellow who told her this joke, her good friend Eulogio Rodriguez, whom I was going to meet. And she was laughing because I would soon have to suffer his jokes myself.

She assured me that the beans were fartproof and, with a final chuckle, began dishing out the chili. She added some sliced tomatoes and bread and butter, and sat down.

"Next time I'll let you try some of my pasta," she said. "Pasta con frijoles, of course."

PART TWO

THE FOUR MOTIONS

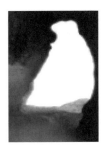

BREATHING

Through movement, through breathing, through the use of the eyes, through voice and language, people interact in a few predetermined dances. This is most notable not for the few steps that are taken but for the multitudes that are left out. I am constantly amazed at the depth to which this choreography reaches, all the way into the very cellular structure of the participants.

—Esmeralda

L ater, we sat in front of a fireplace, which gave off the only light in the room. We both had been gazing into the flames for a while, when Esmeralda spoke.

"Turn around and look at the flickering light in the room," she said.

I swiveled around in my chair and watched the moving shadows play on the white adobe walls.

"Relax," she said.

It felt good after the long day to sit back in that comfortable chair and listen to the night noises. Far off a coyote howled.

Esmeralda began speaking, like a storyteller weaving a tapestry:

"As children we are born living in tones and vibrations. It is as if we are in the midst of a huge orchestra, with countless sensory experiences available. As we get older, this concert is still going on, but we don't realize it because of the way we have been trained.

"Before a baby is born, it doesn't breathe, eat, talk, stand, or walk. Even the vision is unshaped. The pressure inside its body is causing it to grow.

"Now, remember the outer membrane we talked about before? When a baby is born, it trades its amniotic sac for a bigger perceptual membrane. At the moment of its birth, this luminous cell is pliable, resilient, and full of pressure.

"Then it begins to be pressured into certain perceptual agreements by the other cells around it — its family.

"This process can be visualized as a spherical luminous cell being impinged upon by cells of jagged contours, until it adapts to those contours."

I could feel what she was talking about.

"When the baby is in the womb," she continued, "it is surrounded by warmth. That warmth nurtures it. After its birth, the baby looks for that warmth, which we will call affection. In its search for the warmth it once knew, the baby gladly acquiesces to certain perceptual agreements.

"In this time we live in, those perceptual agreements, or ways of grouping together perceptual inputs, predispose a child to certain repetitive patterns. As these perceptual patterns are put in place, they keep the child from experiencing contact with the world in its fullness."

Esmeralda leaned over and took a sip of tea. I did the same. We sat there in silence for awhile. Then she went on.

"It is important that we become aware of and study, on a body level, the mechanics with which our learned behavior is imprinted on us. What we have found is that we can divide the tonal vibrational pressure that molds us into four distinct but very interrelated actions. These are breathing, moving, the use of the eyes, and the making of sounds.

"Let's start with breathing," Esmeralda continued. "Breathing massages our body in a wave. I want you to feel this.

"While you are resting there, you can feel the breath moving through your body. Feel the wave move through your chest and abdomen, all the way out to your fingers and down to your toes, and up into your head and around your eyes. Experience that for a while, until you can feel your whole body expand and collapse as you breathe in and out."

I was surprised that I could feel my breathing all the way out to the tips of my fingers and toes, and in my head, and all over. I focused on my breathing body and, as it expanded and collapsed, I found that my thinking had dissolved. However, I couldn't sustain this state for long before thoughts started intruding.

Esmeralda began to speak again.

"Our thoughts and emotions are reflected in our breath. In many traditions, the breath is often used as an object of meditation, because by watching it, you watch your mind. You can watch the way you cluster and fixate the sensory stimulus of the world. You watch your world come and go, as you breathe in and out. When we get angry, we breathe in a harsh, rough way. When we feel sad, our breathing is very shallow. Every thought and emotion has an accompanying kind of breath.

"Our bodies are constantly talking to each other. One of the ways we actually communicate with each other is through our breathing. When we synchronize our breathing with another person, we are synchronizing ourselves with the tonal wave flowing through their body, including their thoughts and emotions.

"Imagine when you were a baby, just born. You were held on your mother's belly. You were looking for affection. You began to synchronize your breathing with your mother's. In your own way, you emulated her breathing pattern. It made you feel a part of her, like you were before birth. You began to put the world together tonally the way she did. As you began to emulate her breathing wave, you began to make her world view your own. You began to take on the way she clustered and fixated light, the sensory stimulus of the world. After a few months of this, the foundation was set for you to see the world the way she did.

"Most everything else you have learned in life is based on this foundation. You force everything you learn later on in life to fit into this framework."

Esmeralda chuckled.

"Incidentally, most people think that they have free will. But it is only an illusion, because their choices are only choices in the limited world view that they have been conditioned to."

She stopped for a moment, then went on.

"What I am trying to have you become aware of is how deeply we are affected. We are trained very deeply, down to a very minute level, a cellular level of movement that is physical. The limited world view that you have been taught is hitting you from all sides, from the people around you, and penetrating deeply into your being."

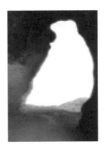

Use of the Eyes

Suddenly Esmeralda stood up, looming over me like I was a child. "Look at me when I'm talking to you!" she said. I automatically turned and looked wide-eyed at her. She laughed.

"The second of the four ways we are molded is through the use of our eyes. We are taught to see in certain patterns. We learn to see ourselves the way that the surrounding breathers see us. Remember your mother picking you up, and looking into your eyes? The energy emanating from her eyes gave you something to focus on. In looking back, you began to parallel and reflect what she saw in you. You molded yourself in her image. In the pressure of her gaze you found the outlines of who you were supposed to be."

Esmeralda began to chuckle as she sat down, bringing my focus back into the room.

"I was just thinking of clusters of cooing women surrounding a new baby, fixating the baby with their hungry gaze," she laughed again. "Wanting someone to emulate them, to justify their existence so they wouldn't feel so alone in the world.

"In fact, this is what we learn to do in day-to-day life. We learn to capture someone's attention and look for agreement in their eye movements. If you really want to get someone to agree with your view of the world, make them look you in the eyes when you're talking to them, and force this agreement on them. It helps!" she chuckled.

"Not knowing how to use our eyes when we are babies," she continued, "we learn to emulate the eye movements of the breathers around us. The options of clustering and fixating they give us are the only ones offered to us. So we adapt. We learn to move our eyes the way that they move theirs, because we want their affection. We learn to differentiate objects the way that they differentiate objects. We learn to categorize things emotionally through our eyes, the way that they categorize things emotionally through their eyes. The eyes actually learn to move in set patterns.

"Let's do some simple exercises. This will be a gross experiment, but it's a good way to have you experience how your learned behavior is imprinted. I want you to feel the way you have been trained.

"Imagine the next time you come to see me, that you're eating a plate of pasta con frijoles." She laughed. "What would it be like?" She chuckled again. "Set the scene up!"

She waited a minute, then asked, "What's it like?"

"Are your eyes directed up, down, sideways?" she asked before I had a chance to reply.

"Looking up," I said.

"Good," she said. "You were imaging the future. Your eyes were looking up.

"Let's try a remembering. Remember the last time you walked down into Huang's studio."

I remembered walking down the staircase and seeing the *bagua* in the brick floor of his studio.

"Are you there?" she asked.

I nodded my head.

"Where are your eyes?" she asked.

"My eyes are looking down," I said.

"Okay. Remembering is looking down. When you see a person who is downcast, they'll be looking down, and remembering or mulling over their predicament in life. If you can make them look up, or focus in any other direction, they will lose that mood. It might be hard, though—they might really want to lick the polish off their shoes!" She laughed.

When I looked up at her again, she was looking at me, her eyes rolling around madly. What kind of joke was she pulling now? I started to laugh. She came up and bopped me on the head.

"Be serious!" she said. "Roll your eyes around and around like this!"

"Okay," I said, and followed suit.

"Now think about your old girlfriend, the one you grieved about for so long."

She chuckled. "One person's torment is another's delight."

"I can't!" I said. I kept trying to picture my girlfriend. "If I keep rolling my eyes, she disappears!"

I began to feel frustrated about not being able to call to mind someone I had been so close to. I stopped rolling my eyes.

"Very good," she said, sitting down. "You see that rolling the eyes, even with the lids closed, makes it difficult to hold or sustain an image."

She reached over and laid her hand upon mine.

"I want you to notice the effect of your eyes on your inner voice and your ability to image. I want you to realize that each of these actions, breathing, the use of the eyes, moving and sound, are interlinked. To explain them I am deliberately pulling them apart. I am giving you these different slices so that you can see them separately and then put them together at the end.

"So, going on with the use of the eyes," she said, "even when you're asleep, your eyes are moving in set patterns, literally in the patterns of your world view. The motions of your eyes are actually creating the images in your dreams and following them, all at the same time. It happens simultaneously.

"You aren't just creating the images or following them, you are living them. Your eyes move when you're dreaming, and there is a reaction in your whole body. Remember waking up from a nightmare feeling exhausted, or from a dream full of animals and iridescent color, feeling exhilarated? Your whole body lives these dreams.

"I'm sure you've watched a sleeping dog twitching and turning its body as it cavorts in a dream world, chasing rabbits." She chuckled.

Esmeralda asked me to put more wood on the fire. I got up and went over to the wood box. I picked up a couple of cedar logs and carefully put them on the fire. When I sat down again, she continued talking.

"Remember the luminous body sac that Huang talked about, and the outer luminous membrane that I talked about?" she asked.

"When we close our eyes, the eye sense goes inside and is actually working with the body sac. During a dream, the perceptual membrane and the body sac are one and the same. When you open your eyes, your perceptions go outward and reflect off the bigger sac."

She stopped for a moment and looked into the fire.

"Dreams try to equalize the way your body sees and the way you have been taught to see. When your body sac and your perceptual luminous membrane are the same, you can see what your body sees, instead of what the learned behavior has taught you to see. Dreams are the result of your natural self, your healing body, trying to contact you in the language closest to what you are used to understanding.

"The eyes move in set patterns," Esmeralda said. "These patterns are learned. The problem is that these patterns restrict the eyes to certain motions, restricting them from the wide range of variables possible."

Esmeralda sat back in her chair and stretched.

I yawned.

"It looks to me like you're about ready to go and see how your eyes move when you sleep," she said. "See you in the morning!"

She got up and left me sitting alone in the room. I turned and stared at the fire for awhile and then went to bed. I didn't know if there would be many dreams left after a day like I had just had.

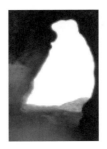

Movement

The next morning I lay in bed for a while, my eyes still closed. Then, as was my habit, I opened one eye and looked around. Maybe that was a signal, for at that moment the door opened and Esmeralda came stumbling in. She seemed drunk.

I didn't know that she drank. I was startled, not knowing how to talk to her. By this time my other eye was open. I wasn't sure how to act. She was making me nervous.

She wobbled and stumbled about the room. I was confused. How should I respond to this intrusion? What was she doing in my room anyway?

Finally, she came up to my bed and sat down. To my surprise, she chuckled.

Then, in her normal voice, she said, "Breakfast is served!"

Abruptly, she got up and walked out of the room as if nothing unusual had happened.

After breakfast we sat relaxing with our warm cups of tea.

"What kind of tea is this?" I asked.

"It doesn't matter," she said. "It's just flavoring for the hot water. I love hot water, don't you?"

That was the opening I'd been waiting for!

"What kind of flavoring did you put in your tea before you came into my room this morning?" I asked.

She laughed.

"Did you enjoy my performance?"

"No," I said. "It made me feel very uncomfortable."

"Well, what made you feel so uncomfortable? Was it something I said?" she asked innocently.

"No, it was something about the way you were moving around, like you were drunk!"

"Oh, that," she said. "Well, how am I supposed to walk? Why don't you get up and show me."

Now I was flustered.

She looked at me, laughing again. "You fell into that one just fine.

"Now we're ready to talk about the third of the four motions: movement. In the same way that we become locked into a way of breathing and into a language of our eyes, we become accustomed to a certain language of movement.

"When you're lying in bed, you don't expect someone to walk in, wobbling like a drunk, telling you the frijoles are ready.

"As we grow, we learn to move. Just as your mother imprints your eyes with her view of the world, the breathers and lookers around you are training you how to move.

"We have a dialogue of motion happening all the time. We set up this action-reaction, stimulus-response interaction with other people through our movements. In the same way that we look for agreement through our eye movements, we also look for agreement in motion. Social interaction is a ritualized dance," she said.

"There is an infinity of training involved in a simple walk down the street. Our joints have very large ranges of motion, but we only operate within a small percentage of that. If you move in a way that people don't expect, you can confuse, frustrate, and even frighten them.

"The way that people learn to move is culturally determined, and people from different cultures can make you feel uneasy, just like a drunk does. They're giving you the wrong cues, not the ones you're used to.

"Usually, black people don't move like white people, or white people like black people, and Indians don't move like either one. This is part of the cause of racial tension. People don't have the same dance, so they don't trust one another."

We each picked up our teacups and took them to the sink. I washed the dishes while Esmeralda dried.

At one point, Esmeralda looked over at me.

"The main way this training is instilled in us as children is through fear; threat of loss of contact and affection, and sometimes physical punishment," she said.

Esmeralda flicked her dishtowel at me.

"You paid a heavy price to buy into that club," she said.

She watched me as I put the dishes away.

"If you know that another person is watching you," she said, "you are going to feel like you have to move the way you've been taught. If you meet someone from a different culture who is talking to your body, using motions that you don't understand, you will respond with the fear instilled in you as a child, just as you did when I walked into your room, moving like a drunk."

I was unclear.

"Why would unfamiliar body motions cause me to be confused and bring up my fear?" I asked.

"Your uncertainty of how to act will remind you of other times that you were uncertain, and take you back to how you were trained to face that uncertainty. Remember that when you were a baby, you were very uncertain how to act in the world of grownups. They taught you how.

"Learned behavior tries to make you feel secure in a specific, limited way. If you deviate from this pattern of behavior, you will be reminded of all the effort that was put into creating it. As I said before, you were trained through fear. This included the fear of losing contact and affection, which is often marked by the fear of physical punishment and other threats.

"When you get into any uncomfortable situation, the foundations of your learned behavior will rise to the surface to be seen, if you're there to watch. Remember that!"

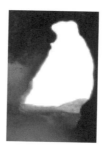

SOUND

It was early afternoon. We were walking along the creek near Esmeralda's house. The canyon walls above us showed red through the bare sycamore branches. Pools of water flowed one into the other. I felt peaceful walking alongside Esmeralda. It amazed me that I felt this way, when I could remember all the times that she had shocked me. Although there was a voice inside of me that was constantly telling me to be on guard, I almost always ignored it. I actually loved being with Esmeralda.

We walked on down the trail until we came to some flat rocks beside a large pool. We sat down in a shaft of sunlight filtering through the branches above. The mood of the place was tranquil, crisp, pristine. We sat for awhile, maybe half an hour, without uttering a word. I absorbed the tranquillity, feeling myself a part of this magical place.

Esmeralda leaned over and spoke softly in my left ear.

"The elders say that the words we speak drop to the ground like stones. But that the sounds we make go on forever."

She sat upright and began to speak. Her voice mirrored the soft sounds of the water moving below:

We live in a world of sound
We are sound

We are singers,
  born into this world to sing our song
The old language speaks with purity
  through the songs of our feelings
resonating from the core
  to fill the vastness of our being.

I didn't understand her, but I knew what she was talking about. Tingles went up and down my spine, the way they did when truth was spoken.

"In the same way that we are taught a pattern of breathing, seeing, and moving that limits our possibilities," she said, "we are also taught a way of speaking and making sounds that is also limited.

"Although different peoples speak different languages, and in doing so isolate themselves to certain physical sounds over others, this is not the most limiting factor that we are taught."

She touched her perineum and her throat at the same time.

"It's more important where your body is resonating from when you speak.

"We are taught to speak in a way that limits the area of our body that we use to resonate sounds in. One of the things we are taught is to talk from our throat rather than from our body cavity. We talk outwardly from our throats, when we could make the sound go down from the throat, fill the cavity of the body, and radiate outwards.

"In this way, we could talk with our whole bodies. Instead, we become more interested in the meanings of the words we are saying, in their cultural context, than in the resonance of the sounds."

She paused and looked at me.

"Proper chanting can allow us to focus vibrational qualities of sounds throughout our body cavity so that our whole body is filled with the sound."

Esmeralda began chanting a very simple chant that sounded like it was in an American Indian language. She motioned for me to join in. As I chanted and felt the sounds vibrate, I tried to focus on what she had said. I noticed that I felt more and more whole, and more and more peaceful as I let the sound resonate and fill me.

"Close your eyes and feel this," she said. "I will move the sound up and down my body."

She continued chanting and I could feel her talking to me tonally with her body. As she moved the sounds up and down her torso, I resonated with them. I began to feel our bodies talking to each other, through sound.

When we stopped, I noticed that the chatter which had been in my mind was no longer there.

We sat in silence for a few minutes. Then she told me she wanted me to try and discover what was behind my breathing, my moving, my normal eye movements, and my internal chatter.

"Good luck!" she said, "I'll see you back at the house when you've solved this problem."

I spent the rest of the day alone addressing the question Esmeralda had left me with: How could I get beyond the imprints of the four motions?

I found that if I walked quickly through an unfamiliar landscape, I could flood my vision. This quieted my mind, but I was still moving and breathing. If I sat still, and closed my eyes, it seemed almost impossible to stop myself from thinking, and I was still breathing. If I sat still, closed my eyes, and focused on my breathing, I found I could quiet my thoughts. But what about my breathing?

At that point, I tried holding my breath, but I couldn't last for very long before the fear in the pit of my belly overwhelmed me.

I couldn't think of any way to quit breathing. Nevertheless I kept trying every way I could think of for a couple hours.

After awhile, I began feeling surrounded, suffocated by the compulsive stimulus coming at me from all sides. If what Esmeralda had been saying was true, there was no way out.

I separated myself from the suffocating feeling enough to allow myself to go over Esmeralda's question again. I thought about what I had done and felt that I had taken all the options I could think of to their logical ends.

I learned long ago that when I truly posed a problem to myself, and followed all of the logical options available, somehow another door would open for more information to come from a place beyond reason. So I did the next thing which came to me. I took a break to allow the answer to come. I never knew where such answers came from.

I stretched and opened my joints. I began walking. I climbed to the top of the canyon and watched the sun set across the big sky.

Before it was totally dark I made my way back to the house, looking for dinner. Little did I know I was cooking tonight.

I wasn't a very good cook, and Esmeralda missed no opportunity to remind me of my shortcomings. She would say, "If you want a New Age woman, you've got to be a New Age man," and she would laugh herself silly, as if it were the funniest thing in the world.

"You'll understand later," she said. "Then you can have a good laugh, remembering!"

"So what did you do this afternoon after I left?" she asked as we sat with our after-dinner tea.

I told her about my efforts to solve the problem she had posed, and where I had ended up. I said that the best I could do was to sit, close my eyes, and focus on my breathing. In certain moments, I was able to put myself in a posture where my eyes were still, I didn't move, and I didn't think, but I could only do that by concentrating on my breathing.

"Great!" she said.

"But I was still concentrating on my breathing," I said.

"Oh, you don't get it," she said smiling. "Who was concentrating on your breathing?"

"I was!" I responded.

She looked at me and giggled.

"Well, who are you?"

PART THREE

THE MALE-FEMALE AGREEMENT

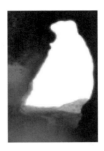

BREAKING THE AGREEMENT

I woke early the next morning. Esmeralda had told me to get a lot of rest. Although I awoke hungry, Esmeralda told me that it was important that I fast until evening. She said that this was going to be an auspicious day for me.

"Just water," she had said. "It's the pure food of the spirit."

I dressed and put on my walking shoes. Esmeralda said we were going to take a little hike. I did a few of the warm-up exercises that Huang had taught me to ease my nervousness and went out into the main room.

Raucous singing was coming from the pantry. Did this woman ever rest? If well-being was a disease, I think Esmeralda had it.

I sat down in a chair facing the fireplace and waited. She came in shortly and wished me well.

"Are you ready to go?" she asked. I nodded, and she went on, "Then let's get packed."

She went over to a corner of the room, and began bringing out some rather large dolls, nearly four feet tall and very solid. I had noticed them standing in that corner before, but had never paid much attention to them.

"These are for you," she said.

"For me?" I asked.

"Had 'em made special," she chuckled.

There were two pairs, each made up of a male and a female figure. One pair was clothed and the other was naked.

The naked male was a stick figure put together from branches of pine, with a peeled branch sticking up for his penis. The trunk of the body of his companion was a curved piece of wood, carved so as to leave two knobs for breasts and a knothole between her spread legs.

The other pair was similarly carved with rudimentary clothing. The man wore white pants and shirt and a hat. The woman wore a skirt, blouse, and a red flower in her hair.

Esmeralda began to tie the two men together and asked me to help her. She warned me not to use those granny knots I tied my shoes with.

"Let me show you a special knot to use," she said. "Go over twice and around once, like this. See, it holds the inner tension really well, and when you want to release it, it is very easy. These knots are going to have to hold for a while."

Next we tied the two women together. We tied these two bundles together and then secured all four figures to a pack frame. The men were on the right, the women on the left.

"These are for you to carry," Esmeralda said as she disappeared into the pantry.

I picked them up. The four dolls together felt like they weighed about forty pounds. I wondered how far I was going to carry them. Esmeralda emerged carrying a small pack.

"Are you ready?" she asked. I shrugged. "Then let's get started," she said as she helped me put the dolls on my back, and we left.

I had been following Esmeralda along a trail for about half an hour when she stopped and signaled for me to pass her. The next thing I knew she was behind me, cackling.

"What is so funny now?" I asked, stopping and turning around. I was trying not to show my irritation. She kept laughing, and motioned for me to turn back around, which I did.

"You look so perfect from this side, carrying that heavy load," she said, catching her breath.

"What's so perfect about it?" I asked, unable to contain my irritation any longer.

"You'll know someday. Hindsight is 20/20!" she said, and burst out laughing again. "I'm not really laughing at you. I'm laughing at myself, and at the world, and remembering what I had to go through. And, I'm laughing at how there is no response for laughter when it comes from the whole body."

We walked for three or four more hours. The trail roughly followed a creek. Sometimes we climbed up from the creek bed and walked in the hot sun on the mesa above. As the hours passed, the dolls got heavier and heavier. I stopped to rest for a moment and asked Esmeralda how far we had to go.

"Are your friends getting heavy?" she asked with a smile.

"Yes, they are," I told her.

"Glad to hear it! Part of the reason we are walking this far is for you to feel how heavy they really are."

We walked for another half an hour, and the land around the creek bed started to level out. A few traces of long-abandoned human habitation began to appear.

Eventually we came to a pole planted in the ground. I saw another one just like it some seventy yards away. They looked like posts used to mark out a country horse-racing track. From there we took what looked like a once well-used trail that branched off to the right and came to a stand of trees around an old, rundown bullring like those I'd seen in small Spanish villages. This one had not been used for many years.

"Well, here we are!" Esmeralda said. "Why don't you drink some water and rest a bit before we go in. It'll be a while before you can rest again." Hearing her talk that way made me nervous.

"What are we going to do?" I asked.

"I'm going to show you something very important," she replied. "I want you to be very attentive. So for now, rest and gather yourself."

After ten minutes Esmeralda stood up and motioned for me to pick up my burden.

"I normally don't like rituals," she said, "but I want you to experience something. I want you to see how your body is affected by the male-female agreement. This is a chance for you to get a taste of your real being."

She walked up to the entrance to the bullring. I followed. Two creaky doors stood ajar, the wood rotting from their hinges. Esmeralda slipped between them easily but had to help me sidle through because of the encumbering load on my back.

I walked out into the circular arena. Here and there weeds grew in the sand.

Even though the stands reaching up around me were falling apart, and most of the paint was gone, I was reminded of the many times I had been to bullrings in Spain and the life and death drama I saw enacted there. I had always been fascinated by the people, the squeamishness of the newcomers, the passionate blood lust in others, and the gleam in the eyes of the old men who came to watch the courage of the bulls, hoping they could get a deeper understanding of their own approaching death.

Esmeralda motioned for me to follow her. She walked along the wall a little ways, then sat with her back against the side of the ring and her knapsack next to her. I took off my heavy pack and started to sit next to her, but she motioned for me not to.

"Now it is time for us to set the scene," she said. "First I want you to find the center of the bullring. Take your time. Make sure you find the exact spot."

I walked out toward the middle of the bullring. A collared lizard darted into a crack in the wooden wall of the ring.

I found what I thought was the center of the ring on my first pass, and put a rock there. Then, from the center, I began pacing to the sides at right angles, forming the arms of a cross. I retraced this cross until I found the center and moved the rock to this point.

"Well done," Esmeralda said from the side of the ring. "Now come here and gather your friends."

I walked over to Esmeralda.

"First untie the knots that you so carefully tied before," she said. "Try and remember how you tied them as you untie them."

Slowly I untied the knots, feeling the ropes move between my fingers, watching the intricate patterns of tension loosen as I worked.

"Now, go and put the naked pair of dolls on either side of your rock," she continued, "on a horizontal axis facing me, with the man on the right and the woman on the left. Start with them about four feet apart, and then adjust them so that when you stand over your rock, you can see them both at once."

I did what she told me, then turned to her.

"Does that feel right?" she asked. "I want them far enough away so that you can feel their presence without feeling cramped, and close enough so that their presence is still powerful."

I went back to the center of the bullring and moved in a straight line between the two figures. I decided to move them a little closer to see if I could feel them better that way. Then I went to the center again and walked back and forth some more. I adjusted the figures three or four times until I could both see and feel them as I moved between them. When I felt satisfied I looked back at Esmeralda.

"Okay," she said, "come back and get the other two and take them to the center," she said.

When I was back at my rock in the center, she directed me to place the clothed figures so that they were the same distance from the first two figures as the first two were from each other, and that same distance back.

"Now," she said, "put your back to me and stand between the two naked figures. The clothed figures should be positioned so that you can choose whether or not to be aware of their presence when you stand in between the two naked figures.

"Walk forward, until you are even with the clothed figures, keeping them in your peripheral vision. Make sure you can still feel the presence of the two naked figures behind you."

I really had to grapple with what she was talking about. But after about ten minutes of concentrating and moving the figures, I got them in the right position.

She then told me to turn around. From this position, no matter how I tried to concentrate on the clothed figures in my peripheral vision, I couldn't ignore the naked backs of the figures in front of me. I said this to Esmeralda.

"That's perfect," she said. "Now come back over here."

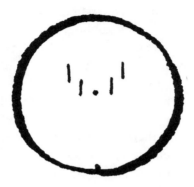

MALE-FEMALE AGREEMENT

"I want you to feel the presence of who was watching you breathe yesterday afternoon. Become the watcher."

I walked over to where she was sitting.

"Sit in front of me, facing the figures," she said.

I sat about a foot in front of her. The change in her voice had signaled me to move into a new mood of serious concentration. I began to relax and became aware of the ground beneath me.

We sat there for a while. The movement in my body quieted. I stretched my vision by separating my eyes to the sides. I watched the breathing wave flow over my body. As my breathing stilled, I felt glimpses of being the watcher between the waves of conceptualizing thoughts.

Raucous magpies flew around in the trees circling the bullring, squawking at the figures I had set up. I began to realize how much concentration it took to see through the eyes of the watcher.

A voice behind me broke the silence.

"The linchpin of the training we receive from the other bodies around us, through their breathing, looking, moving, and talking, is the male-female agreement. The nature of this agreement is the basis of our societal structure. It is what creates our society.

"The male-female agreement of a particular time is what delineates which aspects of our creative powers are made available to us,"

Esmeralda said. "Society's fear of the creative power within each of us has placed tremendous restrictions on its expression.

"These restrictions mean we are allowed to move only in certain habitual patterns. The patterns greatly limit the arranging of stimuli, or the ways that our inner being can contact the outside.

"When we start to pull the energy back from our habitual actions, this loosens the knots that our society has around our creative power. It is like a person standing bound with knotted ropes. If the person compresses inward, all of the ropes will fall off his body to the ground. Then the person can learn to spread the compressed energy back through his body and learn to move again, without the binding ropes of convention.

"This compression is actually a gravitational realignment between heaven and earth. We pull the energy that has been absorbed into a repetitive relationship with the outer world back into ourselves. We reestablish our connection with heaven and earth.

"When the connection with the spirit has been reestablished, we must learn to let it flow through our body. Like babies, we have to learn to move, but this time without the encumbrance and reinforcement of knots about us. We have to learn to move from a neutral place, not a place that is defined by the negative-positive polarities of our learned behavior.

"The way to reach the spirit, in the midst of the polarity of our learned behavior, is neutrality. Neutrality, in terms of our learned behavior, is the beginning of more options. It is the beginning of more contact, contact that is not bound by society's restrictions.

"The part of you that has been watching yourself breathe is the closest you can come right now to this neutrality. Moving around in the world, while being in this position of neutrality, is the way to begin to allow volition to move in your being in new ways.

"Now I want you to experience the movement of volition," Esmeralda said. "Stand up slowly. Remain concentrated as you move. Don't turn around. Put your weight evenly on both feet while you face the figures."

I filled my body with the awareness I had gathered and began to stand in this new way. I could feel my old way of standing creeping in. A great deal of concentration was required for me to stay neutral, and to neither act nor react in the manner my usual way of standing was demanding.

"Now bring that sense of the observer into the standing posture. Spread it through your body with pressure, as Huang taught you. Energize your body with it. Let volition—your luminous essence—fill you."

I stood there, legs bent as if riding a horse, with my wrists pushing down at navel height. In this position, I created more pressure and interconnected my body with that pressure. I felt my feet begin to push into the ground. This downward pressure began to create an upward pressure in my arms, which felt like they wanted to rise. I didn't yield to this, but held my arms in position, and this increased the overall pressure even more. I maintained this posture as best I could with my attention on this internal pressure.

I held this position for a few minutes.

"Now I want you to move," Esmeralda said, "to walk the way Huang showed you. Walk slowly, deliberately, with pure concentration. Walk to the first pair of figures and stand between them."

I began to move slowly, keeping my body concentrated and pressurized. One foot up, one foot down, I carefully walked forward. It seemed like an eternity. Awareness flowed through my body, allowing more and more minute levels of movement to become conscious. Finally I was standing over my spot in the center of the ring. I could see the male doll peripherally on my right, the female on the left. Maintaining contact with these two figures through my peripheral vision stilled my mind. Behind me, I could hear Esmeralda's voice.

"Concentrate on the two figures on either side of you."

Esmeralda paused for a moment, then continued.

"Now I want you to go down deep inside of yourself, and determine what the core is of what you've learned is female," she said. "Then, likewise, feel the core of what you have been taught is male."

I went inside myself. Time slowed. Vision opened. I was very surprised by what I found. What I saw was a frightened young girl. She stood with her arms wrapped around herself, almost cringing as if she expected a blow. She was frozen, and there was a black and blue cast about her, as if her circulation was poor. I felt that she was so fragile that any noise or movement might shatter her.

On my right was a young boy surrounded by a dull brown, reddish glow. He was stomping around like a lumberjack. He seemed totally insensitive, knocking things over, and rather dumb.

Both the girl and the boy were innocent in nature. There was no way to judge them. They simply were. I transferred these feelings onto the naked figures. This seemed inappropriate because I had found children, and these figures were sexually mature.

Then a strange thing happened. My images and feelings of the children and the figures merged, and I understood that the sexual images I had been given were basically those of children, even though my learned behavior had confused me into applying these patterns to the adult men and women around me.

Esmeralda seemed to know when I had transferred my male and female energies to these figures, for she started talking again.

"Now I am going to explain to you how you are stuck in your perception of the world. It's as if there's a powerful pressure pushing your face up against a molded windowpane. You can't turn your head, because you don't even know that possibility exists!

"Stay neutral. Keep your being focused on the male figure to your right and the female figure to your left. Keep your feelings merged with these figures.

"It is the male-female agreement that is the source of the pressure pushing your face against the window. This relationship, between the living images that you have been taught, is the linchpin of your belief structure. That's what you found waiting for you within yourself."

Esmeralda stopped. I felt the silence all around me. After a moment, she continued.

"Now, as you stand there, aware of the figures on either side of you, focus on the two clothed figures in front of you. The two figures on your right are the male-male agreement. The two on your left are the female-female agreement. These are the beginning of the extension of the male-female agreement into the social contract. The male-male agreement and the female-female agreement both support, and are supported by, the male-female agreement.

"Feel how males interact with each other, and how females interact with each other. Let images flow. See how these agreements create, and are created by, the male-female agreement."

I focused first on the two male figures on my right. I wrestled with a sudden influx of memories and feelings. They surrounded me, all clamoring to speak, to have a voice. I struggled to make them somehow intelligible. Faces and scenes quickly came and went. Finally I managed to still them until an image could form.

I was in the seventh grade, twelve years old. A bigger boy was threatening to beat me up. I sized him up and didn't think I had a chance. I was afraid. There was a wrenching feeling in my chest as I tried to figure out how to back down without losing my sense of being a man.

The memory dissolved and another image took shape. An older boy was threatening my younger brother. I felt obligated to help him, but I didn't know how. I was afraid of having to face the older boy.

That picture in turn swept away. I refocused on the two male figures. Then pictures arose of my friends in childhood, the alliances I had struck up in order to have someone to be with. I played sports with them. With our games we danced a ritual that would bind us together and protect us from the violence all around.

Older boys telling crude jokes about women. I saw again the looks on their faces, the feeling that there was something looming ahead that I needed to know about.

Sitting around playing poker in smoky rooms. Talking about sports as a way to feel comfortable around other men. The images went on and on. I started to touch the walls of fear and pain that had made me into what I had learned a man was supposed to be.

I looked then at the two female figures on my left. When I focused on them, new images flooded through my mind. They tumbled over each other, images that had been transferred to me from women I had known and feelings that had come to me from observing women together.

At first they were just a blur, feelings and experiences from the past filtering through me. After a while there seemed to be a residue that I could look at. Something that linked them all together surfaced. I found I didn't feel as closely aligned as I was with the male figures. It was an interaction that I was only indirectly involved in.

It was a woman's world. Here I was an observer, not a participant. However, I could arrive at its basic premises from the mirrored male-male agreement. I could sense the basic agreement among women, an agreement which defines their actions with one another and with men. Even as I sensed this, a series of images came forward to hold my attention.

The images swept past like the landscape flowing around a train. They began with a very striking woman who I knew, an aerobics instructor and belly dancer, telling me about a student of hers, a woman in her early twenties who was the most beautiful woman she had ever known. My friend was telling me that the beauty of this woman made her feel insecure. That image was replaced by one of the same friend a couple of weeks later, her face radiant. "You know that student? She came to me and told me she was pregnant! She didn't know what to do! But I got the whole story out of her. The boyfriend is from a wealthy family, and she thinks she likes him. I told her it was obvious, get married and you'd be set for life!"

I had listened to her in disbelief as she gave me this glowing account of the wonderful thing she had done.

The train switched tracks. New scenery. A new series of images began to flow by, set in a beauty parlor. An older woman, a middle-aged woman, and a young woman, are sitting under hairdryers in the haze of chemical smells from newly curled hair. They are giggling and laughing. The older women are talking to each other, complaining about the problems in their marriages. At the same time, they're ribbing the younger one about when she is going to get married, to join the club, so they can go to the wedding.

I was interrupted by a voice.

"Now slowly move forward until you can see the clothed figures out of the corners of your eyes. At the same time stay very aware of the naked pair of figures behind you."

I walked forward slowly, concentrating on keeping the images behind me alive, until I was even with the two clothed figures.

85

"Now I want you to extend your awareness to the grandstand in front of you," Esmeralda said. "Fill them with people. Gather all the feelings you have experienced with the male/male, female/female, and male/female agreements. Feel these agreements spreading outward until they fill the world, forming the social contract."

As I stood there, aware of the figures around me, I suddenly felt suffocated. It was the same feeling I had as a kid around grownups. I had felt like a prisoner, smothered and controlled.

Then a memory surfaced of a summer picnic that I went to with my family. The men were barbecuing the meat and playing horseshoes, talking politics and money. I somehow felt they were suffocated, too, trying to enjoy these events because they thought they were supposed to.

I watched the women putting out the tablecloths and plastic forks, complimenting each other on the food they'd brought and asking for recipes. I could feel the male-female agreement behind me, flowing through the male/male and female/female agreements to create a sense of community.

I noticed that among the people at the picnic there seemed to be a hierarchy. Those who were higher up and got their way a lot seemed to be more comfortable. Everyone seemed to be vying for the little bit of comfort that was available in this limited system. It was very suffocating for me to watch them feed off each other. I felt better just being a kid.

Then I saw the little girls running around the picnic tables. I didn't want anything to do with them, and yet I sensed that they were really just as confused as I was.

I felt terrible. I felt forced into watching, absorbing, and learning to partake in this ritual. How you give, when you give, why you give, is the ritual, acted out in a physical choreography, an energetic representation of the male-female agreement.

As I looked around at the people at the picnic, I saw them in "stocks"—those wooden things people used to be locked into, to shame them into social compliance. The men and women at the picnic were plastered into limited ways of acting, with limited body movements. It was as if they moved with plastic body plates in front of them, and the

86

children were being herded into the body plates of learned behavior being passed down to them through their parents.

Watching the men, the women, the children, I imagined them waking each morning and fitting into their body plates. After a while, they got so used to fitting into their body plates, that they believed that's who they were.

"Now I want you to turn around," Esmeralda's voice came softly as the images began to fade. "I want you to imagine pulling your face and body away from that body plate."

I began to slowly turn to my right. She stopped me.

"No, you usually turn that way. Turn to your left."

As I complied, I suddenly felt myself ripping away from something. It was as if the whole front of my body had been glued to a molded piece of transparent plastic. As I turned, I felt myself separating from this plastic, the glue that bound me stretching thin, then finally giving way, bit by bit.

It was hard to turn around. A very strong current was pushing against my back, trying to keep me faced toward the grandstands, pressed into the plastic shield. As I slowly fought my way around, I felt that the very core of my being had shifted loose. The pressure of the current was a waterfall whose roar filled my ears. All of the feelings and images that had been summoned up seemed to be pushing against me. It was hard to maintain myself, my neutrality.

"There is a way through this," Esmeralda said. "At first it will seem like a thin line in the middle of it. Concentrate the pressure in your body. Fill your body with volition, with light, the way Huang showed you."

Suddenly I could see a path open for me in the midst of that current. I slowly began to walk. When my energy wavered, Esmeralda reminded me to walk carefully, deliberately, and exactly. I finally made it to the two naked figures.

"Rest for a bit here," she said. "Gather your energy."

"You are in a very special place," she continued. "This is the doorway between worlds. When you move beyond this point, you will be plunged into the world of the basic two, self and other."

Esmeralda stood up, picked up her knapsack, never taking her eyes off me. She walked a little ways to her left and opened the bag. She pulled out four iridescent parrot feathers and laid them down on the ground pointing in the four directions, brightly colored against the sand. She removed a gourd rattle with angular crimson designs painted around it, and then a rabbit's foot. She placed these on the ground as well.

She went to the right, about as far as the two clothed figures were from each other. She pulled out a Bible, a rosary, and a picture of a Hindu master. She then returned to her spot at the side of the bullring.

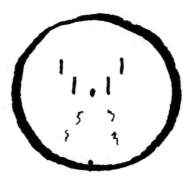

SELF AND OTHER

"Now you've come to the difficult area," she said. "The area of psychism, sorcery, and religion is the world of self and other. This world is even more dangerous because here there is so little definition between you and your reflection. Here you are face to face with your mirror image. It is in this region that your idea of who you are interacts with its shadow.

"It is very difficult to walk the road of neutrality here, because as you go down this path, there are jewels that glitter on the side of the road. The temptation to stop and pick them up is overwhelming. It will get harder and harder as you go further, but you must resist. For if you leave the road, you will disappear into the mists of glamour and illusion."

As I walked towards Esmeralda, I had to concentrate on putting pressure in my body and feeling my feet.

Images and feelings came to me of when I was younger, in college, when I had started to feel new energy rising within me. I had not known what to do with it. I felt ripped apart. I'd wander the streets at night, in the city where I lived. Occasionally, I would go into a church and stare at the statues. These statues would often talk to me. I couldn't remember what they said. That hadn't seemed important. What was significant was that I could live in a world where Jesus and the Virgin talked to me.

As I slowly stepped forward, new images rushed into my mind of friends who had been distraught about the state of the world. I saw how they looked for a way out through spiritual paths and ritualistic practices, and yet they continued to define themselves in the same way.

I could see their faces. The same expressions. They hadn't really changed. They had never faced the core issue of self and other. They just took their new spiritual concepts and adapted them to their old idea of themselves and their bodies. I felt sad thinking of one particular close friend because, to this day, she seems no closer to a fuller expression of herself than she did back then. Like so many others, she managed to change clothes, but still lived in the same body of her learned behavior.

I remembered my feet again. I may have experienced all of those images in the time it took for me to take one step. I didn't know.

I continued walking. Finally I stood in front of Esmeralda. She was still sitting against the wall.

She looked up at me, and said, "I sit in the middle, and I am your teacher now. I give you the presence of my body, the foundation, the power of my speech, and the conscious awareness of my mind."

She told me to turn around, this time to my right.

"You have to walk back down the path, recreate yourself. Go back through the land of power, mystery, psychism, and religion. Go back through the male/female agreement, back out to the social contract."

She paused and then continued.

"Now that you have a feeling for how you have given up your power, and a feeling for who you really are, you have to go back through your recreation to reclaim yourself.

"What is important is the road.

"Your body.

"The place where you are stepping."

I began walking and Esmeralda gave me much of the same instructions that she had given before. She told me to walk slowly and deliberately, connected to the earth. She made me aware that it was important to reexperience self and other, the male-female agreement, the male-male and female-female agreements, and the social contract.

I felt my learned behavior as an hourglass constricted in the middle by the male-female agreement. I walked back and forth for I don't know how long.

Gradually, I felt more neutral, comfortable and relaxed. Between the sides of the hourglass that I had constructed, I began to embody the feeling of neutrality. The path I was walking on broadened, and the sides of the hourglass drew apart.

Time stood still.

At one point, while I was walking towards her, Esmeralda told me to stop between the naked figures and gather myself.

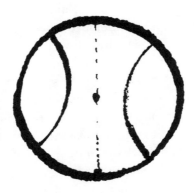

HOURGLASS

I stood there for a long time.

The shadows of the trees covered half the bullring when Esmeralda told me to come towards her. She handed me a box of *cerrillos*, Mexican wax matches.

"Gather together the two naked figures and the two clothed figures," she said, looking into my eyes. "Go to the side of the bullring and pull a sliver of wood off the side of one of the grandstands. Pile these on your spot in the middle of the ring. Gather the objects of power and mystery in the realm of self and other and arrange these as kindling. Do this slowly and carefully, remembering the feelings that each of these evoked."

This took awhile. The experiences I had just relived had shaken the foundations of my ideas about myself.

On the one hand, I felt very fuzzy and disoriented in terms of my old way of seeing myself. On the other hand, I felt very clear and precise, and in the present. In the midst of this split, I could feel a swell of life and emotion beginning to surface.

After I piled everything carefully, Esmeralda said, "Remember that I am here behind you as you set them on fire."

I slowed my breathing. I carefully lit the match with one strike, and looked at the flame move through the paper. I watched the flame spread, setting the pile on fire. I turned slowly and walked back to where Esmeralda was sitting.

I sat in front of her, watching the pile burn. I felt very tired. Looking at the fire and listening to it was very soothing. Esmeralda didn't say a word.

When the fire finally died, and the last smoke had blown away, I heard Esmeralda stir behind me. She reached around me with both arms and laid a spade on my left side and a small sack on my right.

Put a little sand in the bottom of the sack, then put the ashes in it," she said. "You need to take care of them properly."

I got up, walked over to the ashes, and scooped them into the bag. Esmeralda got up and signaled for me to follow her out of the bullring.

When we got back out to the trees, where we had rested earlier that day, she told me to go and find a place to bury the ashes.

As I walked into the trees, I didn't quite know where I was going. I felt a bit wobbly. I stumbled around until I found a place that felt right.

I dug a hole and buried the ashes. Then I placed the paper bag on top and lit it on fire.

I went back to where Esmeralda was. She led the way to a nearby road. She told me we were going to have to hitchhike back.

As we stood by the roadside, the desert sun painted colors all around us as it set below the horizon.

After a while an old white pickup appeared in front of us. A longhaired woman in her early thirties rolled down her window. Esmeralda began talking to her, telling her our destination. The woman turned and talked to the longhaired man who was driving and also tried to quiet the two noisy children who were squirming between them.

When Esmeralda and the woman spoke, and then the man and the woman, I watched between the hellos, the talking and negotiating, and the glances down at the children to keep them in check. I watched the choreography of their family ritual. I felt the agreements that bound them together and understood the feelings of suffocation that made the children squirm. Having reexperienced these things myself, I knew what they were feeling.

The woman told Esmeralda they'd give us a ride. We climbed into the back of the truck and settled down, with our backs against the rear of the cab. It was wonderful to sit under the stars, watching the scenery recede.

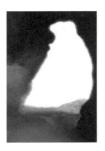

THE PRESSURE OF AFFECTION

When I woke up late the next morning, I felt peaceful. I went out into the kitchen to find some breakfast. Esmeralda was nowhere to be seen.

The walls of the rooms seemed different. Somehow there was more space between them. Colors were more brilliant. Memories surfaced and passed away, like leaves falling on slowly flowing water. A veil had been rent, and I was living in a new, expanded world.

I spent the morning quietly, listening to the swallows under the eaves outside.

Esmeralda came in shortly after noon. She asked me if I was hungry.

"We always have *frijolitos* here," she said as she began pulling food out from cupboards and off of shelves.

Before I knew it, I was sitting down in front of a scrumptious meal. There was thick venison stew poured over rice, a dark green salad, cheese, and bread. For dessert we enjoyed truly delicious persimmons. I found myself rubbing my face into one, sucking it into my mouth. It was the most sensual food I had ever eaten.

"Let's go for a walk," Esmeralda said after we had finished, and I had washed my face.

Soon we were in the canyon again, walking through a crunch of dry leaves. Occasionally, a bird chirped overhead. The pools of water had a stark beauty, slowly flowing one into another, yet seeming not to move at all. The canyon walls were both warm and severe. I became intoxicated by the smell of fermenting leaves all around me.

We walked on, step after step, pool after pool. I could feel myself open to the sky.

We came to a place with comfortable rocks by the water and sat down. It was midafternoon. The winter sun was delicious, nurturing, soothing, and warm. I liked looking at the rushes, the brown rushes on the sides of the pool, rustling in the soft breeze like crickets rubbing their legs together.

Esmeralda started talking.

"When you relaxed into the neutral zone you found yesterday, you were freed from being pulled by the forces of your limited view of reality into either a negative or positive alignment with them. You were able to recall your light. This allowed the spirit time to create new ways of making contact with the world. As you continue to expand, your limited view of reality will cease to exist the way it used to.

"Remember, your body is a slide, a photographic transparency." she went on. "The spirit shines through your body and is projected out onto the outer luminous membrane. Your habitual actions have made wrinkles form in your luminous cell, decreasing the surface through which you can contact the world.

"When you relax into neutrality, an alignment is created with the body that knows."

Esmeralda paused for a moment.

"You were coerced into giving away your natural alignment through the sympathy agreements you made with the other humans around you. Now you need to realign yourself, get back the energy you have lost, and refocus it back out into the world in new ways."

"How did I get coerced into giving my energy away in the first place?" I asked.

"You wanted affection," Esmeralda said.

"Is there something wrong with looking for affection?" I asked.

"No! True affection, true contact, is what we are all looking for. Honestly needing to exchange energy with others is important. Acknowledging the contact that we need from one another forms the basis of our interaction. Our work is in discovering who we are and where our true affection lies."

I was confused.

"What does affection have to do with alignment?" I asked.

"When we are babies, we are naturally aligned with gravity," she replied. "We have a lot of natural pressure. We have a lot of resilience. Since we were recently in the womb, we have a very direct experience with affection, or the sense of being connected with everything around us.

"After we are born, we are looking for that kind of contact again. We are closest to having it as babies because then we are still naturally lined up and full of pressure. We begin to lose pressure because of the agreements we are forced to make and repeat over and over again in order to make contact with other human beings.

"We are surrounded by beings involved in the male-female agreement of the particular time and culture. We are taught that there are only a few circumscribed ways of giving and taking affection.

"If men and women aren't supposed to be in this male-female agreement, which in turn creates the social contract and causes all these problems, what are we supposed to do?" I asked. "How are we supposed to act?"

"You have to remember," Esmeralda said, "that relating isn't the problem. The problem is the way that we relate. The male-female agreement that we live in now is very limited. Our potential as human beings is therefore hampered.

"The elders say that if people are true to their own nature, and are not afraid of their own nature, a whole new way of relating is possible." She stopped for a moment, and went into deep thought.

After awhile, she said, "I need all of your attention now for what I am going to say."

"The affection that you now can perceive is just the stepping stone for something greater, a greater affection."

Once again, the way that Esmeralda said that made tingles run up and down my spine. I could feel the truth in her voice. My body knew she was right, but my rational mind somehow didn't have the capacity to grasp what she was saying.

Esmeralda looked at me and smiled.

"This is very difficult," she said. "It takes a lot of energy to understand this. It will take even more to incorporate it." She laughed.

"Well, let's at least try and play with the understanding of it.

"The spirit is sitting on us like a hen on her eggs, waiting for us to hatch. We are in the process of forming inside of these eggs. We don't know where we came from, or where we're going, or what we will be when we get there. In fact, all that our individuality is, is a glance at the inside of our shell.

"We come out of the womb looking for that warm affection that we have lost. We become lost in the illusion of self and other. Then we are trained to contort our natural being in order to gain just the tiniest bit of that affection. We are caught in the pincers of the male-female agreement, and the resultant social contracts. Most people stay stuck at this level.

"If you were to proceed to look for the source of your affection, looking for the root of your desires, a gate would open and a path would appear. Then, as you fill your being with affection, you will realize that there is something beyond.

"This is the pressure of affection, the pressure of light that begins to dissolve the shell of our learned behavior. The pressure from the inside begins to feel the affection from the outside, and the shell gives way.

"We are the affection that is created by the merging of the spirit within us into the greater spirit that is eternally waiting out there."

Esmeralda fell silent and we sat listening to the water and the rushes moving in the breeze. Wafts of intoxicating smells from the fermenting leaves were interspersed with the dry sounds of birds busily rustling in the undergrowth.

I was infused with a warm glow that met and fused with the gentle winter sunlight. I felt full.

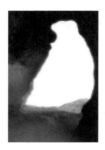

CELESTIAL PIVOT

A couple of days later I was driving down towards the Mexican border to meet with Eulogio, whom both Esmeralda and Huang referred to as their "little brother." Huang had given me a package to bring to him. Esmeralda had given me two.

As I drove, I thought about a conversation Esmeralda and I had shortly before I left. We were in the living room, talking about the male-female agreement and the experience in the bullring. I felt that certain things had happened to me that I understood, but could not voice. I was sitting there, groping, asking the best questions I could.

"Enough of this talking," Esmeralda said suddenly. "Stand up."

I stood up.

"Walk back and forth across the room," she said. "Keep talking.

"Often, being in the sitting posture, things can get stuck," Esmeralda continued. "If we begin to walk, a new circulation of energy happens.

"I want you to talk as you walk. Let things move. Get some clarity and flow from changing to a moving posture."

After five or ten minutes of walking, and what I thought was mumbling on my part, Esmeralda said, "That's better. Now stand still and face the wall."

The next thing I felt was Esmeralda's back against mine.

"You're not going to kick me again, are you?" I asked.

"Naaah, we've already been through that," she chuckled. "But I do want you to remember that experience. Slowly turn around, like we did before, but this time we are going to be more specific." We began turning. I could feel Esmeralda's back against mine. As we turned, she spoke.

"Feel again how the majority of your sensory egg is in front of you. Most of the ways that you sense the world are in the front part of the body. Our training has to do with manipulating our sensory inputs, and most of that training is stored in this part of our body. This is where most of the filters of our training reside. From now on, let's call these filters 'shields.' They protect us from the onslaughts of undifferentiated energies, and they also keep us from experiencing them. It's the loosening up and manipulation of these shields that our work is about."

When we stopped turning, and were facing each other, Esmeralda put her hands on my chest.

"In here are housed the solid organs," Esmeralda said. "They are deep storehouses of memory that need protection.

"That's why we have ribs," she said as she poked me.

Then she moved her hands down to my abdomen, placing them on either side of my navel.

"Down here in the abdomen are the functional organs, sometimes called hollow organs. In them food is digested and transformed into energy. Strengthening this area is a key component of our work." She started to move her hands downward from my navel.

I jumped back. She chuckled, and then continued.

"In this area is the root and storehouse of the life force that runs our body."

She motioned for me to come right up next to her again. She noticed that I was uncomfortable standing like this.

"Make pressure in your abdomen like Huang taught you, like you did in the bullring," she said. "Fill your abdomen, then drive the energy into the ground." I did this and felt myself relax.

"Its time to tell you about something else," Esmeralda said, as she stepped away.

She motioned for me to sit down. She went over to her bookshelf and pulled a picture out of a large book. She walked back over and placed it on the table in front of us. It was a beautiful picture of a baby inside the womb. I could see the umbilical cord connected to the sac around it.

"Originally we had an amniotic sac," she said. "When we were born, we lost that. It is through that sac that we make a direct connection with the world around us. That original sac goes away at birth, but we are still connected to the world through this area of the body."

She leaned over and touched my navel.

"We still are nourished from this place, and it is here that we store what we've learned about differentiating energies. All kinds of energies!"

She sat back in her chair and continued.

"As babies, when we start to eat and receive input from the people around us, our immune systems develop. We learn how to digest food. We learn a certain way of differentiating between what is 'good' for us and what isn't. We learn to accept what is supposedly 'good', and react against what is 'bad'. This differentiation is what the immune system is all about, and what makes something acceptable or not.

"At the same time, our psychic-emotional immune system develops. We learn from the people around us what are acceptable ways of interacting with people, and what are not. We do a great deal of this learning about differentiation, of both physical and emotional input, in the first three months of our life. It could truly be said that during this time the foundation is laid for what comes later."

She paused and then added, "The creation of our shields or world view thus begins."

"What about the four motions we talked about earlier?" I asked.

"Like I told you then," Esmeralda responded, "this process of acculturation is many-faceted. What we talked about before mostly involved the physical communication mechanisms that are used to imprint the social contract of the time onto a child.

"Now, we are talking about where it is stored. Think about

when you feel overwhelmed. You will often feel nauseous. Remember when we were standing facing each other, how nervous you felt? And when you calmed this area," she said putting her hand on my navel region, "it settled you down.

"The point that I am trying to make is that this area, the abdomen, the area around the navel, is where both our physical and emotional immune systems develop, the immune system being that which differentiates what we believe is good for us from what we believe is bad.

"What you are doing now is working with loosening and manipulating your shields so that you can regain the contact with the outer world that you had when we were young.

"The so-called physical body is a key. If you make a change in your idea of the physical body by allowing more of the spirit to flow through it, and then you stabilize that change, you create a permanent difference in the range of possibilities that are open to you. It's no longer just a little excursion into a possibility of how to make contact with the world out there in a new way. It becomes a stabilized reality."

She paused and then continued.

"But you already know about that. From your work with Huang, you've started to feel that if you change the body sac, the projections on the outer luminous cell change, too. He has shown you that by creating pressure, aligning yourself with gravity and thus allowing more energy to flow through you, you can make more contact with the world around you."

Again, I was driving. I noticed my hands on the wheel, the desert passing by, the clear blue sky above. But my memories were too enticing, so I returned to them.

"If you create a habit of more pressure, you can stabilize a new level of energy," Esmeralda continued. "The first object of our work is to ignite the spirit. We want to have it, our luminous essence, flow into the physical body, and then out to affect the rest of our world. If you can maintain this pressure, the body can store more and more light. This stabilization of light then creates a platform for even more of our spirit to move through us.

"What we want to do is to have the spirit, our luminous essence, move through the body, out through the relating body, and affect how we make contact with the world.

"Therefore, as the spirit begins to inhabit more of our body, and more of our relating body, the neutral zone that you just experienced becomes greater. The neutral zone is any place in between our learned behavior.

"What you are learning will allow the spirit to flow in a bigger environment. The luminous essence from the inside of the body is allowed to merge with the energy on the outside of our being, and makes more contact with the infinite waves of energy that are out there."

My recall was shattered by the sight of what appeared to be a couple of ravens around a roadkill. As I got closer, the birds got bigger, and I realized that it was a pair of spotted eagles. In awe, I watched them as they took off, each massive wing-beat created a rush of air that vibrated through the surrounding land. I pulled over to watch them rise and circle.

Then, high off to the right, a third eagle appeared. It plummeted toward the first two. It hurled itself at one of them, and they rolled over and over, screeching. They separated just as suddenly. It was inspiring to watch them and, before I knew it, they had disappeared up into the sky.

Getting out of my truck, I walked over to a fence post. Rusty old wire was hanging to the ground. The relief of emptying my bladder was immense.

While I stood there, watching the parched desert ground soak up this moisture, a wall fell inside of me. I remembered something else that Esmeralda had said about the abdomen.

"The elders say that everything in the area above the navel is ruled by heaven, and everything below is ruled by earth. The place where these two energies intersect is the birth of man's energy and everything he creates. They call it the celestial pivot.

"When we look at our habitual patterns carefully, we see that the make-up of our shields centers around fear and loathing of the earthly energies. These are the downward flowing energies of urination, defecation, and sexuality.

"The male-female agreement is the way we have been taught to perceive this area below our navel. Because this lower abdominal area is the source of creative energy for our body, it has great significance. When we begin to release the restrictions in this area, we allow the energy to flow more unimpededly through our whole body."

Thinking back on this, I remembered how Esmeralda had warned me not to get too caught up in the idea of the male-female agreement.

"Remember," she had said, "the male-female agreement has practical value because it is a very functional way to clarify our experience and relate it back to our body slide.

"It's efficient, it gives us a good overview, and it's even fun," she had said, chuckling. "But the male-female agreement is still only a means to an end. What we're really after is gaining energy."

I had smiled at her and rubbed my belly.

"Gaining energy, in turn, enables us to make more contact with the waves of the world at large." She had laughed and rubbed her belly, too.

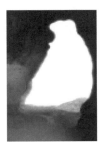

WATCHING THE AGREEMENT

My journey to visit Eulogio continued. It was late afternoon when I pulled into a small town near the border. I parked in front of a little restaurant and walked in through a pair of swinging wooden doors. There was a row of red vinyl booths on either side of the room, three on the left and four on the right. Past the booths was a counter with a cash register at one end. Adjacent to the counter were a couple of tables beneath windows facing onto the street. It was the kind of place a retiring couple might set up, after dreaming of having an ice cream parlor and then realizing they needed to sell burgers and fries to make ends meet.

An old man and woman appeared on cue. I looked at the menu and thought fondly of Esmeralda's *frijoles*. The proprietress came over to my table to take my order. As she stood there, a group of pubescent girls came in with a flurry of shrieks and giggles. They descended into one of the booths on the far side of the restaurant. I placed my order and watched them.

They must have just gotten out of school. Notebooks and pencils covered the tabletop. One girl was scribbling notes, another with a new hairband was being fussed over. In the same high tones, the group began teasing the girl who had been scribbling notes about some boy.

Suddenly a motion caused me look to my left. I saw a boy's nose pressed against the outside of the window. From my first startled impression of his nose I went on to see a freckled face, a baseball hat, and a group of boys standing on the street behind. The girls saw them too, and their voices got even louder as they pointedly looked away.

One of the boys in the group nudged the boy with the baseball hat, and he took his face away from the window. Before I knew it the whole group came banging in through the swinging doors and settled into one of the booths on the right side of the restaurant across from the girls.

The elderly lady set my food down in front of me. As I ate, I watched the show. Sitting here eating, my perspective began to shift.

The scene in front of me transformed. Instead of girls and boys, I saw energy moving back and forth between luminous cells of light.

I looked over at the knowing expression the old couple behind the counter shared with each other, and I knew that they had been seeing this same scene for years.

I watched the energy of the kids moving back and forth. It was difficult to see these children as individuals. They seemed rather to fit into groups of cells that were interacting with each other. The boy who had put his face against the window, and the girl who had been scribbling notes, seemed to be the focal point from which the energy sprung.

The enormous energy of youth that they had was suddenly coming face to face, body to body, with the male-female agreement.

They were unsure, shy, testing the water in groups. As the boys threw spitballs at the girls, and the girls giggled, laughed, tried to ignore them, sending the energy back, I began to clearly see the choreography of the ritual they were playing out then and would continue to act out through their lives.

There was a motion at the door, and my eyes were drawn away by the sight of the same patterns just forming in these children, but now fully shaped. A young couple had just walked in and sat down at the booth behind the young girls. They were looking into each other's eyes.

While the kids were under the suffocating energies of the male-female agreement, and trying to learn about the social contract it implied, these people had been molded by it, as if fitting themselves into a body condom. They danced the ritual of the time without hesitation. However, they were already losing the bursts of energy that the kids shot off like fireworks.

Suddenly, my view was blocked by a slow, depleted, dull light. It was the same pattern I had been observing in the children and young adults, but it was worn out. My vision shifted. I shook my head. I looked up and saw the elderly woman standing in front of me. It seemed to take all of her energy just to smile at me as she put the check down.

I wondered how many pharmaceutical drugs she was on, how many of her organs had been removed. I wondered how she really felt about having paid the price of participating in that ritual.

I left some money on the table and stood up. I remembered to create pressure in my body as Huang had taught me. I relaxed and walked past the counter where the old couple leaned. I walked slowly and deliberately between the confused and exuberant energies of the kids. I walked by the young couple sitting near the door and, although I felt their eyes reach out to grab me, I maintained my place of neutrality.

I swung the doors open and smelled the crisp air of a desert winter evening.

PART FOUR

LUMINOUS BODIES OF LIGHT

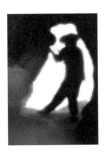

REFLEXIONES:
THE PATH OF A HEALER

I have been very fortunate to be in the healing profession.
Being a healer has kept me very close to the pulse of life. It
has given me a place from which to observe the play of life
and death in the body. It has presented me with very real situations in which to put my theories into practice and to see what
value they may have. It has also allowed me to probe the depths
of a question that has great importance to me: What is a real
cure?

The path of the healer has shown me that real medicine is
the study of well-being, not the study of disease. I have learned
that the focus in medicine should be on preserving life and wholeness. I have seen very clearly that studying disease and forgetting about the rest of our being causes confusion, and that studying life creates unity and clarity.

In my practice, I have noticed that the process of healing
involves focusing on a Bigger Dream, something beyond our
normal self-concept. This change of focus alters the way we deal
with the world and allows us access to a greater spectrum of
energy. My task in healing has become to reconnect people to
this Bigger Dream, and the core of my diagnostic procedure has

been to perceive what is keeping that connection from being made.

What first led me to the path of healing was wanting to know, for very personal reasons, how my emotional states related to my physical body and the diseases that this particular relationship would predispose me to. I studied whatever I could find to help me understand this dynamic. I found that there was not very much information available because our cultural view of the body is very limited. It was very difficult for me to explore sensations that were beyond our cultural framework, beyond our words.

The multisensual body models of shamanistic healing and Chinese medicine helped a great deal. Chinese medicine's 2500-year written history gave me perspective on how our idea of the body has changed through time. It showed me that the idea of the body is a fluid and changeable concept. For example, in old Chinese medical thinking, the body had a more direct connection to the physical elements of the world than it does for us now.

The Chinese model and the models of shamanistic healing have given me rich and vibrant alternative ways of seeing myself and others. Many ancient models see the intellect as a sense, like seeing, hearing, touching, smelling. From this I've realized that the perceptual mix of our time highly stresses the mental and visual aspects of our being. To move beyond this stress, I've been inspired to feel and explore reality in ways other than the mental-visual cultural framework within which I grew up. In doing so, I have discovered a whole body cosmology based on a multisensual reality.

These studies have allowed me to learn much about the nature of perception. To a great degree, mental-visual sensations create past and future, while the other senses, such as touch, taste, smelling, hearing, have a sense of time which is more present, mysterious, and magical.

Shamanistic healing and Chinese medicine have provided metaphors that have allowed me to go beyond my cultural matrix, to feel movement and flow in my body and to give this sense of flow importance. This sense of flow has given me other identities to juxtapose with my learned behavior so that I can slip in-between and around it.

Using the path of the healer as a vehicle for moving beyond my learned behavior has been very challenging. When I first started, it seemed as if I were going nowhere. But something inside of me kept pushing me on. I didn't know why. My learned behavior was always questioning, always asking me, "What are you doing?" and "Is this producing any practical results?" Then one day, after pursuing this path of "nonlearning" for years, I realized that I had something.

I found acupuncture and Chinese medicine to be very complementary to my study of body movement. When I looked at acupuncture closely, I found that it was really a most precise way of manipulating the force of gravity and how it flowed through our bodies. The most important acupuncture points are located in areas of maximum articulation on our joints and torso. Ultimately, acupuncture has to do with the movement of our joints and how we use movement to pump energy through our bodies.

I also began to notice, in myself and others, how the sensual consensus that we grow up with can cause many diseases. Often, in a very few moments, I would get to know people as well as if I had known them for years. Through this process, I saw how, hidden in our family values, were generations of lies that make us sick. At the same time, I observed that there is an innate knowledge within the body that, when called upon, can heal us. Not only can this inner knowledge, our luminous essence, heal us in a physical way, but it can give our being direction in embodying a state of well-being or completeness.

The study of gravity and body mechanics gave me a very immediate methodology to follow, something very practical to do in the present. The male-female agreement and the strategic perspective it offered allowed me to see how I progressed through time. And lastly, the study of shamanistic and Chinese medicine and disease, through my own body and in my clinic, provided a theoretical container with its multisensual body models—a proving ground for my theories.

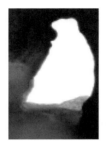

EULOGIO THE HEALER

The ways of perception I see people around me choosing make up a very limited and repetitive choreography when compared to the rich iridescent tapestry of possibilities available to us as humans. These limited and repetitive patterns create tendencies towards certain diseases.

However, because we have within us a healing body that knows—a knowing body—we need not be confined to these repetitive perceptual inputs that predictably make us sick and limit our life span.

—Eulogio

I always enjoyed driving in the desert. It seemed so bleak at first, yet after entering into it for a few days, I could feel how full of life it was. Being on a vast expanse of land allowed my mind to expand up into the clear sky. My mind felt clean.

I took me two days to drive slowly down to the border town where Eulogio lived. I crossed the border in the early evening.

For me Mexico always has a certain smell. I don't know if it is the tamales, corn husks, or marketplaces, but it always makes me feel comfortable, as if somehow I've returned to a long-forgotten place that I know so well. Mexico is for me a place where life is not hidden. Everything is out on the street: children, beggars, couples, and families, raw meat hanging in the market.

I remembered once staying in a small town in central Mexico which I ended up calling "The Village that Never Slept." I had been hospitably put up by some Indian friends, only to be kept up all night. First it was the roosters that never seemed to sleep, and then the screams of a pig next door. This pig must have been butchered very slowly, for I could have sworn it squealed from two to four in the morning. Of course the children were up at five. To this day, I don't know why those roosters never slept.

Eulogio lived in an older part of town, full of big trees, splashes of color from the Mexican flowers, and the smell of the river.

I knocked on the front door. It was opened by a man of medium height, with beautiful almond-shaped eyes and dark curly hair. He seemed to be just a little bit older than I was. He smiled at me with a Cheshire grin. I introduced myself. He laughed a little and seemed genuinely glad to see me.

I put out my hand, and he lightly touched my fingers, the way the Indians in Mexico often greet each other. He said, in a very soft voice, "*Eulogio Rodriguez, a sus ordenes.*"

I responded to the traditional Mexican greeting in my less than perfect Spanish, and he said, "I see. Let's speak English. At least most of the time."

He smiled and asked me if I would like to come in.

"I brought some presents for you from Huang and Esmeralda," I said. "They're out in the car."

"Oh, them?" he said with a knowing laugh, his eyes lighting up. "You'll have to tell me how those old guys are anyway. Let's go get those presents, and your things."

We brought my bags into the house, and he showed me around. We went through a corridor into a courtyard with many doors. The house was U-shaped, the two wings connected by a high wall with huge trees bending over it in the back. All parts of the house opened into the central courtyard. In the middle of the courtyard, near the back wall, was a fountain that looked like a natural rock spring. Water gurgled out, seemingly for the enjoyment of the abundant population of birds. There was a table with comfortable chairs by the fountain, and hammocks hanging from a couple of mid-sized trees in one corner.

As Eulogio took me to my room, I noticed a kitchen, a laundry room, and other bedrooms. The massive old walls gave a sense of weight, stability, and peace to the place. The air, even this late in the year, was laden with the scents of flowers and moist, fertile earth.

After I had unpacked and washed up, I strolled out into the courtyard. Eulogio was sitting by the fountain, on one of the comfortable chairs by the table. He stood up graciously and asked if I was hungry.

"Not really," I replied.

He sat down and motioned for me to do the same. He asked me about Esmeralda and Huang and told me to thank them next time I saw them for the things they had sent. I told him that, in talking to them, I had heard a lot about him. But no one would ever tell me how he got his first name, Eulogio. I had never heard that name before.

"Oh, that," he chuckled, then said with a smile, "Which story should I tell you?"

"The real one," I said.

His belly shook with laughter.

"My mother said that, when I was born, she didn't know what to call me. There were some strange birds outside making a chortling noise, almost under their breath, a sound like 'ee-u-lo-gio, ee-u-lo-gio.' And being the woman that she was, she decided that should be my name. Eulogio, at your service!" He stood up and took a bow.

I shook my head, thinking, "Not another one of these characters."

He began asking me questions about where I had studied healing, where I had traveled, if I had been to China, my ideas about the body. I found that I began to relax in his presence. Just talking to him, the tension in my shoulders and the weariness of long hours of driving fell away. Somehow I felt at home. I told him how relaxed I felt.

"You're just noticing the results of my work," he said. "It took years for Esmeralda and Huang to turn me around. Each day, I am more and more in awe of what they did for me. I can't even remember my world the way it used to be. I will be forever grateful for the doors they opened for me. You're a lucky man to have drawn them into your life."

He seemed to listen to the fountain for a minute. Then he inhaled some of the fragrant air and said, "How about now? Are you hungry? I am!"

He stood up and I followed him into the kitchen.

After eating, he mentioned that he had a few things to do, and told me he would see me in the morning.

Early the next morning, I came out of my room to find him doing exercises in the courtyard. I assumed they were exercises that Huang had taught him, but they weren't familiar to me. After a bit he waved me over and asked me to show him what Huang had taught me.

Although Huang had taught me many movements, the majority of my teaching from him had centered around a certain series that he called the "form." I showed this to Eulogio. This form took approximately half an hour to do.

Eulogio watched very carefully with great concentration. This had a dual effect on me. It seemed to increase my focus, and at the same time melt away my sense of self. I had more energy in my movement, but I hadn't integrated this energy into the form yet, so I felt uncoordinated. Huang had taught me to keep going when this happened. It meant that I was gathering energy, putting new awareness into my movement.

Huang had told me that the feeling of losing my confidence in this situation was a sign that learning was taking place on a very deep level, and that I was shifting levels of awareness. He had often advised me to carefully observe this process of shifting, so that I could become better acquainted with its stages and relax into them.

When I had completed the form, Eulogio moved closer to me.

"Let me teach you one that we can do together, so that while you are here we can be in the same movement," he said.

"But the only person I've worked with has been Huang, and

he's always shown me the same movements," I objected. "Will learning something new interfere with what Huang is teaching me?"

He waved my words away. "The principles of body motion and the body's relation to gravity, when studied carefully, can be applied in a great variety of ways. The point is to learn the principles.

"The body has an integrity that everyone experiences. Even though what Huang taught you and what I am showing you seem different, it's the same body working with the same principles. So I'm sure Huang won't mind if I change your routine a little." Eulogio laughed to himself. "In fact, he taught me what I'm going to show you. He also taught me that what's more important than the movements is the study of body mechanics."

When Eulogio talked to me about these things, it was much different than talking to Huang, who just showed me things, but didn't actually explain very much. Eulogio's mind was different. His explanations added a great deal to my sense of confidence and direction about what I had already learned from Huang.

After we had finished, Eulogio mentioned that it was important for a healer to do this kind of exercise daily. "By doing this," he said, "the body can be kept strong enough to be able to withstand the force of other people's pain."

After a few days, falling into Eulogio's routine was very comfortable. I found myself enjoying doing these exercises with him early in the morning as part of a daily routine. It was much easier than getting up the energy to do them in a concentrated way by myself.

Walking to the office where Eulogio saw his patients, perhaps half a mile, became a favorite part of my time there. It was a transition between the inner work at his house and the outer work at his office, a place where there was no object of concentration. Everything was allowed to flow without focus. Sometimes I would look down at the ground, sometimes I would pay attention to the way a certain part of my body moved. Sometimes I would admire the flowers in the trees, or listen to the birds, or watch people. Walking with Eulogio had the feeling of flowing down a river.

Eulogio would often ask me about my dreams as we walked.

Occasionally we would stop and sit on a bench and talk about them to share and give our dream life an awareness in our daily life.

When we were walking, Eulogio's mind seemed to be working from a place that was focused, yet diffused. He was open to the possibilities around him, collecting energy from a wide variety of inputs.

Our luminous cells were in motion together. There was a natural exchange of energy between us that went on regardless of whether we talked or not. It brought a great joy to me to be around someone who gave me something of the same feeling as Huang or Esmeralda, but in a normal, daily setting.

I found a different kind of intimacy and exchange with Eulogio than I could with Huang or Esmeralda. I understood that there was something to be gained through interaction with someone with whom I felt on more of an equal footing. There was an ease from having had the same teachers and being able to talk about their teachings without the confrontation of the student-teacher relationship itself. It was also interesting to hear his observations about them. At one point, we laughed for a long time at his impersonations of Huang and Esmeralda telling jokes to themselves.

Each morning, we would get into the office and organize everything needed for the day; then people would start to arrive. The first day I was amazed by the transformation in Eulogio. I watched him put the learning stored in his body into action. He was gracious, charming, funny, able to flow and yet stay direct with whatever came through the door. He became someone who could maintain the pressure of very close contact with people and still function efficiently in the midst of it all.

On the one hand it seemed as if he were always startling people with his infinite variety of jokes and inane songs, and then suddenly he would become very serious. It seemed to keep everyone off balance and yet flowing. In a way Eulogio's life reminded me of a river and its different moods. If the house were the still pool, and the walk between like a smooth current, the office had the energy of a cataract, air and water and rock mixing together exuberantly in sparkling sunlight.

The first day I was there, he said, "There's only one rule: I want you to have fun, and learn, but stay out of my way." I found this to be a consuming task in itself. He treated people in four different rooms at once, going from one to another. He was surrounded by students who answered the phone and did various tasks, patients coming and going, and people who had stopped by to say hello—a regular hub of activity with him in the center.

Part of my time was spent up front with a student. I answered the phone, talked on a variety of subjects to the people who came in and out, and generally enjoyed myself. I noticed that people seemed very different after having spent a little time with Eulogio. Sometimes he would call me in to one of the rooms to ask my opinion on a particular problem. Often I would just follow him from room to room and watch him work.

The patients varied: old and young, men and women, rich and poor, Americans, Mexicans, and an occasional European. Even the gardener who took care of the grounds would come in now and then to see what was going on. The thing they all seemed to have in common was their connection to Eulogio. I marveled at how the spirit flowed through him.

The first morning he introduced me to a stunningly beautiful American patient named Michelle. He put us into one of his rooms and asked for my opinion of her condition. She came to his office almost everyday. Eulogio always managed to find a way to have me spend some time with her, either alone or with him. This must have been intentional, because many of our conversations outside of the office revolved around her.

Michelle was meticulously dressed and groomed. Her expensive clothes were tailored to fit snugly, showing off her large breasts and small hips. Her smile and makeup were flawless. All in all, she seemed to be a perfect model of feminine beauty.

The image she embodied was directed towards creating a specific response, and I was definitely affected by it. Yet, in her presence, I felt split, like I was talking to two different people. One was a very seductive woman, the perfect product of a fashion magazine culture.

The other was a frightened young girl, much like the one I had experienced in the bullring. The first was brittle and in control. The second, although frightened, seemed like she held keys to many other worlds.

That first day I felt very uncomfortable around her. I had related to "Barbie dolls" before, but what I found interesting in her was that she had this other dimension. Her hard plastic exterior seemed to be malfunctioning and letting a rich softness through. This softness would lead me to expose a vulnerable side of myself, and then I would be buffeted about when she responded with the rote responses her image afforded.

Once, when Eulogio and I were walking back to his house, we sat down on a bench to enjoy the sound of water running through a fountain. He asked me what I thought of Michelle. I explained to him how I felt jerked around by the contradiction between her hard outer shell and her inner softness.

"That's good," he said. "She's not very smooth at all. She's split, in a limbo state. Her shields have been broken and they are full of holes. She doesn't have the strength or will to repair them, and she is desperately afraid of engaging the world without them. Sometimes people come to me like this. The spirit leads them here."

He stopped. We watched the *paleta* man wheel his cart by, yelling his guttural vending call. These *paleta* men could be seen everywhere. They wandered around, pushing their carts full of the assorted popsicles called *paletas*. Some of these were coconut, some lemon or pineapple, made from either a milk or water base.

Eulogio started laughing. He told me was thinking about a friend of his who was going to write a book called *The Paleta Mysteries*. His friend saw the *paleta* men as an underground communication system of higher consciousness, spreading itself through Mexico with popsicles. The images of *paleta* men that rose in my mind made me laugh with him.

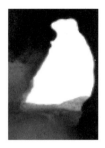

SICKNESS: A CROSSROADS

One evening we were talking in Eulogio's room, sitting in front of a small *chiminea*, or fireplace. We often spent long hours in front of the fireplace, talking. The flames seemed to soothe Eulogio and give him inspiration.

We sat in silence for a while, watching the flames lick the logs. Eulogio looked over at me, looked back at the fire, and began talking.

"Michelle is at a crossroads," he said. "Her shields have been rent. She no longer has the strength to hold her shields together, but neither does she have any other way of expressing herself except through them. She is in a very uncomfortable place! Because of the work you have already done, you have the resiliency to be able to feel this.

"Even though the position Michelle finds herself in is very disorienting for her, it is the beginning place, a place where amazing things can happen."

Looking back at my own experience, I remembered that those times which seemed most overwhelming to me were, in retrospect, the times when I was creating a foundation for new ways of being in the world.

"She is at the portal of a magical universe," he continued, "but doesn't yet have the strength to let the light from that place fill her and express itself through her. It is a very dangerous, yet potent, place to be."

He stopped, as he often did, and looked deeply into the fire.

"At first," he began, "gathering the energy to use her natural instincts to create a new life seems a monumental task. Imagine a spider, just beginning to make a web." Eulogio moved his hands through the air.

"In the beginning, there is just empty space. The spider has to climb up and find a twig, lower itself down, find the edge of a brick. It may even fall all the way down to the ground in order to continue its work."

With the light of the fire upon him, and the motions of his hands, Eulogio brought this picture to life. "Then it has to scurry up a piece of board, and then hook itself onto the drainpipe. What courage and instinct this takes!"

Identifying with the spider, I remembered how I had had to trust my own instinct, and what courage it had taken for me to proceed.

"After the original cornerposts are in place, the web is easier and easier to spin," Eulogio continued.

As I watched him, I could almost feel the sense of completion the spider must have had after manifesting its innate nature in the midst of the void.

Eulogio sat back.

"Michelle has to first pull back from the behaviors that tax her energy," he continued. "This will allow her to regroup and gain strength. Then she can gain the perspective to examine the learned behaviors that she is hooked into, and free herself from them. This will allow her focus to shift away from them so that her energy is available for something else."

I remembered being in the bullring with Esmeralda, and the incredible amount of focus and concentration it took for me to turn my head around and face the energies that had shaped me. I realized how much energy it takes to face one's learned behavior. This made me appreciate even more the things I had learned from Huang and Esmeralda.

"Like the spider, Michelle has to face the void and direct herself to set up a first point in the midst of that vastness out there," Eulogio continued, spreading his hands in front of his face. "Her battle is then to keep going.

"To keep concentrating energy on that point requires great courage. At first, there is very little feeling of accomplishment, or of having done anything. This is the most difficult part. At this point, she has nothing to guide her except for a slender connection with the spirit inside, like the instinct of the spider, and that connection is at first very tenuous. All I can do as a healer is lend her the strength to continue on, to help her to turn around and face the void."

The realization hit me of how difficult it is to start out in a new direction, without any context whatsoever. In frustration, I asked Eulogio why it was difficult? Why can't we just decide to change, and change right then?

Eulogio smiled, and was silent for a moment, listening to the crackle of the fire.

"The more we understand about the vastness out there, the more we realize the fragility of the human condition. Even more so, the fragility of our human conditioning," he said, turning to look at me.

He looked back at the fire for a moment, then continued.

"Our shields are formed through the male-female agreement and our social contracts. They allow us to function socially. However, this social functioning and its conditioned way of seeing things are only a very small portion of who we are. Esmeralda and Huang have taught you about this in their own ways. I am going to show you how this limiting of our potential actually causes accidents, sickness, and disease."

I thought to myself: Are accidents actually caused by the way we've been trained to be in the world?

I gazed into the fire for a moment and missed Eulogio's next sentence. When I came back, he was talking.

"Our being is not satisfied with limitation. The spirit within us seeks to unite with the huge currents outside the luminous cell of our being. These huge undulating waves are like an aurora borealis. They

123

surround us and seek to move through our being all the time."

I watched Eulogio as he stopped to sip his tea. The shadows of the fire played over his body. For just a second, I saw him as a tiny speck in the midst of this ocean of bright iridescent lights. His voice had changed in quality from the rather dry tone with which he had begun. It was the voice of a man speaking to his beloved, full of desire and passion.

"We are floating in an ocean of great waves and currents swirling all around us. Our luminous essence trembles to make contact with its enormous counterpart."

He fell silent. We watched the fire together for a few minutes.

"Although our shields allow us to interact socially, or horizontally, with other beings," he continued, "we forget that there are other ways of making contact with that great unspeakable Other. In this forgetting, our shields become brittle and all-consuming."

Eulogio's words made me remember the people at the picnic from my childhood that I had experienced with Esmeralda in the bullring. I recalled how stuck they were in their body plates, or wooden stocks, and how much energy it took me, even under Esmeralda's direction, to begin pulling away from my limited view of the world.

Eulogio rose, stirred the fire with a stick, and put a few more pieces of wood on fire.

"The spirit is always seeking contact," Eulogio said, looking over at me. "The spirit inside of us will try to find a way to bring about more connection with the world at large.

"We can look at our whole life in this context. What we experience in our lives is really the spirit trying to make contact with the ocean of energy all around us," Eulogio said, as he walked back and forth in front of the fire, his hands clasped behind him.

"Each of us has a slightly different learned behavior, so that what we experience will be slightly different. The nature of the events will depend upon our particular training." He stopped walking, looked at me, and said, "So, you could say that one's training, or one's learned behavior, as it resides in the body, will predetermine our future. We just dance the same dance over and over, until we wear ourselves out."

As I tried to comprehend what Eulogio was saying, the image of the elderly lady who owned the diner came into my mind.

Eulogio walked back to his chair and sat down.

I looked at him curiously. "Is what you're talking about the same thing Esmeralda was referring to when she told me about the spirit as a light inside, the body as a slide, and how it determines our projected image of ourselves?" I asked.

"Yes," he responded. "And what I'm describing takes that metaphor one step further. It puts it into motion—into time and space."

"In what ways does the spirit try and bring about more contact?" I asked.

"Our luminous essence seeks to merge with its counterpart, the Great Other," he said. "In the process of flowing, it erodes away the limitations of our learned behavior. Of course, our learned behavior resists."

I nodded, acknowledging how resistant I had been, and still was. However, at least now I knew that I was resistant and could laugh at myself, at least a little.

"Let's take a look at this from the spirit's point of view." He looked at me and chuckled.

"The spirit first begins with gentle persuasion. People or episodes that will allow us to contact the world more fully are called into our lives. If we fail to respond, then the spirit uses its medium-range missiles." His eyes twinkled.

"These are more like emotional upsets, problems at work; basically situations that require a little more attention. They distract us from our habitual patterns, creating a situation which demands new movement. But we are people, hard-headed and slow to learn," he said, shaking his head.

"If the gentle reminders and the medium range missiles fail to get our attention, then the heavy artillery is called in. Sickness, disease, accidents. These will really grab our attention and disorient us from our limited approaches to life. It puts on the line our idea of what we think our body is and what we believe to be its function in the world. We are forced to relate to the world differently. But people are slow to listen and let the world in."

I thought about how hard it had been for me to learn. I recalled how my life required that I go from one disaster to another before I finally was willing to let go enough to realize that there must be some other way.

Thinking of my experience, I asked, "And what then, if people don't listen?"

He looked at me curiously and said, "And if we still don't listen, the spirit will call on its ultimate weapon—death."

We sat for a while longer looking at the fire.

I began to think about what my role as a healer could be if, as Eulogio was saying, the spirit was responsible for both disease and its cure.

"If illnesses are the result of the efforts of the spirit to help some-one make contact, what is my role as a healer?" I asked.

He turned, looked at me, and said, "It is to help a person's spirit contact the Great Other more and more often, and in different ways, creating a sense of well-being. As healers, we can assist this process, make it more efficient, and allow it to happen without too much dam-age to the body.

"Sickness is a crossroads, a potential opening," he said. "One can either seek to put the body back into its old patterns, or use it as an opportunity to understand the language of the spirit." He ran his hand through his hair, then continued.

"What we often see, in so-called medicine and healing, are ways of patching up holes in the sympathy agreements and social contracts so that people can keep functioning in the same old way. This, of course, only keeps people from listening to the voice of their spirit, and ups the ante."

I thought for a moment. "So, are the people out there who seem to not have sicknesses or problems, closer to the spirit?" I asked.

"Often the opposite is true, and it takes keen perception to see through this," Eulogio said.

"Usually the social conditioning of these people is highly func-tional. Their ability to move within the world of social contracts is refined, so they do very well within them. This allows them to get more energy than most people from their horizontal interactions.

126

"They wonder less about their conditioning because it seems to work so well for them," Eulogio continued. "They are on top of the social pyramid, so they have no motivation for seeking anything beyond their learned behavior. They are lulled into complacency by the way that they have been trained.

"I call this the 'myth of the nurtured child.' You know those children who are raised in the so-called 'right way.' These people seemingly have all their needs met within the confines of their training and find little need to explore the immensity of their being."

He looked back at the flames, and continued.

"These people often don't realize that something is missing until it is too late. By the time they do realize that something is missing, most of their energy is being used up by their habitual patterns, and they have very little energy left to turn their lives around.

"The spirit is always there, rapping, waiting," he said, knocking with his knuckles on an imaginary door in front of him.

"But if one doesn't put his ear out to listen, the contact cannot be made."

"So what about people who are not raised in the so-called 'right way'?" I asked.

"Those people who don't fit in very well are in a better position to be aware of the innate inadequacies in the social contracts of the time," he said. "Since the social contract doesn't work well for them, it is easier for these people to look elsewhere."

"People who have the qualities that the current male-female agreement calls desirable are more entrenched," Eulogio said. "Take Michelle, for example. She's beautiful and appealing within the male-female agreement of this time. This means that Michelle and people like her have more invested in this agreement than your average Jane or Joe.

"They have more to gain from it than an undesirable person. They get more energy from both the males and the females around them because the males and females around them are all trained to support that agreement. But the end result is that these highly conditioned people limit their ways of relating in the world to an even narrower band than an average person."

He stopped for a moment to let the fire fill him again, then continued.

"Because Michelle limited her options in relating, she had less energy at her disposal. This made her very lazy in the eyes of the spirit. So, in order for her to change, the spirit had to hit her very hard," he said.

"Is that why Michelle is in such a dilemma?" I asked.

Eulogio looked at me and said, "When the shields are rent in such a way that it has taken a huge toll on the energy of the body, there is really no more patching them up."

"What rips apart the shield in such a destructive way?" I asked.

"This can happen through situations which severely disrupt the functioning of the shields," he said. "Drug abuse, alcoholism, illness, severe fright, extreme sadness, shock, excessive fasting, improper use of psychic faculties are a few examples."

"I thought we were trying to break down our shields," I said, confused.

"I agree, it's confusing," he said, chuckling. "And it will remain that way unless you begin to see things from the perspective of the spirit.

"The breaking down of the shields is desirable, but it should be done gradually and deliberately in order to maintain ballast," he continued.

"Spiritual paths are basically methods for maintaining this ballast while allowing the shields to dissolve slowly," he said.

"Totally rending the shields, without a strategy, is very dangerous. A person who has done this no longer has the strength to maintain their old agreements, yet a new way of acting or accessing the world has not yet developed. They find themselves lost, without direction.

"They are at a crossroads, in a 'limbo-world.' The old ways of functioning no longer work, but these people can't function in a new way yet, either."

He got up and again began pacing back and forth in front of the fire, hands behind his back.

"What happens to people in this 'limbo world' is that they get sick," he went on, "because their old idea of the body is no longer available to them, and they haven't yet developed a new way to dialogue with the immense world out there," he said. "They become unable to give expression to the forces they have activated internally, and their old ways of being don't have the strength to contain all the new energy they are being exposed to.

"Their circuitry has been blown. They need a new, fluid, energetic model of reality, and it hasn't had a chance to develop.

"They're in a real fix," he said, looking at me.

"What can these people do?" I asked.

"Usually, people in this situation," he replied, "will attempt to pull away from the pressure of relating put on them by the male-female agreement and the social contracts. This will make them feel better for a time because they are not being reminded of how they are supposed to be. And it's appropriate to pause, to give the spirit a chance to move through one's being in new ways.

"But, most people don't take advantage of that pause," he continued, "because they don't use it to create a strategy for dealing with the world when they face it again.

"So, when they do interact with their old surroundings again, they are pulled to respond in their old ways.

"Their shields have deteriorated so that they no longer provide protection. In fact, putting energy into these shields, which no longer operate efficiently, actually wastes their energy and makes these people weaker. Thus, when they make contact with their family and friends, they get sick. This leaves them very confused and directionless."

A sweet smell wafted through the room. Eulogio asked if I wanted to go outside and take a walk around the garden.

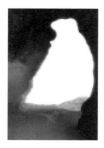

Seeing The Spirit

The next day I saw Michelle again. After having talked to Eulogio, I saw that a lot of the confusion that I had felt in her presence wasn't mine. The confusion had been a result of our close proximity, the merging of our luminous cells, and my inability to perceive the situation clearly.

Now, I noticed that, if I maintained the pressure in my body, I could actually dispel the sense of confusion that I had felt before. I also noticed that, because our luminous cells were merged, the internal pressure that I sustained in my body also relaxed Michelle.

I began asking Michelle about her life before she came to see Eulogio.

She confessed that she had lived a very fast life of money, men, and drugs.

I asked her why she had chosen to live this way.

"I did it just to get away," she replied. "I just couldn't stand my family."

She went on to say that, at one point, no matter how much she liked escaping in this way, her body could no longer take the strain.

"I felt I had to get away from my family," she said. "I just knew there had to be something else.

"Maybe I was wrong, but Eulogio says that my impulse was

right. He says I just did it wrong, too rashly and wildly, and so I injured myself."

She looked at me, and said, "Eulogio says, if I trust him, or at least try some of the things he suggests, I may be able to create a new life and that, with discipline and direction, I can find what I was really looking for—another way to be."

I asked her if she liked coming to the office.

"I like coming here very much," she said. "I feel like I can be myself here. But then I have to go back."

"Go back to what?" I asked.

"My family, my friends, my old boyfriend calling . . . . I just want to go somewhere and be alone."

"How do you feel when you're alone?" I asked.

"Oh, I like it!" she said. "If I can be alone for a day or two, a lot of my pain goes away. But when I have be around my family again, I get sick."

She paused and reflected. "When I come here, I feel better again. I really like the people here."

Just then, Eulogio walked in singing, with a slight Spanish accent, his rendition of an old Southern song, "She was trying to run all night . . . . she was trying to run all day . . . . Doo-dah, doo-dah!"

Both Michelle and I smiled, and the seriousness of our conversation was replaced with his bubbling exuberance.

He asked her about her pain. He examined her, told a joke or two, and had her lie back. Eulogio then placed acupuncture needles up and down her body.

"We always treat the big pattern," he told me. "Then add points for whatever symptoms she's feeling today." He stepped back from the table.

"Did you do those things with your family that I suggested?" he asked Michelle. "Were you able to be more natural around them?"

I noticed that Michelle had relaxed. She was no longer trying to shield herself. The brittleness I had felt in her before was gone. Since she was now relaxed and soft, a new type of concentration was possible, and she was able to respond directly from that richer place.

"Maybe I can spend a little while longer with them before I get sick," she replied. "But I don't like it."

"Remember, it's just relaxing," Eulogio said. "Were you able to interact with them in the way that we talked about yesterday?"

"Well, I gave my mom those flowers like you suggested," Michelle said. "That really changed her for a minute. Then she asked me where I got them, and how much I paid for them. I paused and relaxed for a moment. Then I told her, 'I love you too much to tell you,' and she was pleasant a little longer!

"But when she started talking about how much prettier the flowers were at the store she'd been to, and how low the price was there, I really couldn't take it any longer."

"What did you do then?" Eulogio asked.

"I went back to my room fast!" Michelle said.

"At least you were able to trip up the usual pattern and relax a little more," Eulogio said.

"Remember, we all live in an electromagnetic world, where we're wired to respond to each other in certain ways, along predictable circuits. You're a special case, however. In your situation, your circuitry no longer serves you. In fact, it makes you sick. You can't use it or get caught up in it any longer. The only way out is to begin to discover and use new ways of relating to the world.

"In learning to relax, you are also learning to act in new ways," he said. "This is one of the ways to cure your illness and move on."

When we were walking back to his house, Eulogio asked me what I felt around Michelle this time.

I stopped and told him that when I was with her this time, I had a little more awareness. I didn't get confused like I had before. Also, I told him that I had noticed that when he put the needles in she didn't seem so split.

"Those needles can work wonders in reconfiguring the circuitry of the body," he said.

I then looked at him quizzically and said, "What was all the stuff about the flowers?"

"We'll talk about that later," he said, walking on.

"Well, then what's with the jokes?" I persisted. "And those

songs!"

He laughed, then launched into the old show tune, "Old Man River."

After a few bars, he stopped singing. "People want to convince you that they're sick," Eulogio said. "They want you to think seriously that they're sick! My job is to teach them that they're not sick!"

"How does your terrible repertoire of songs and jokes do that?" I teased.

"You don't like my songs?" he said, as if offended. He laughed. "I thought everybody liked my songs! Maybe I don't sing them loud enough. Is that it?"

I shook my head. I couldn't keep from chuckling myself.

Eulogio went on, "I laugh and have fun to change their electromagnetic pattern. That way, with at least one person with whom they have shared their deepest, darkest secrets, they no longer feel a need to bemoan their fate. In fact, I don't let them.

"They can talk about all those seemingly terrible problems and realize that there is more to life, that each magical moment is a new creation. In this way, they begin to relax into who they are, and realize that there are other ways of contacting the world."

We walked through the park a little further, until we came to a fountain surrounded by benches. There were a few other people there. We sat down and looked up at the trees.

I began to notice the people around us. There was a woman sitting on one of the benches watching her two children play in the fountain. A couple of schoolgirls talked together, still wearing their uniforms.

I asked Eulogio, "You're a healer. Do you see people's diseases when you look at them?"

"Well, you'd think so, wouldn't you?" he responded, turning to look at the children. "But I don't live in the world of disease. I live in the world of the spirit. My world is full of brilliance." He breathed deeply, rolled his eyes up into his head, and laughed.

"I see the spirit in people," he went on. "Disease happens when the spirit doesn't flow. I look at people and see where the spirit flows through them. I think about the spirit and not about disease. And I see how the learned behavior of the times constricts the spirit and makes people sick."

I gestured with my head at one of the children. "Well, what do you see when you look at him through the eye of the spirit?"

"He's young and still full of spirit," Eulogio said.

"What about those schoolgirls?"

"The learned behavior of the times is just starting to get ahold of them. They still have a lot of spirit."

An old man slowly walked by. "What about him?" I asked.

Instead of answering, he sang.

"He's tired of living, and afraid of dying, oh doo-dah day."

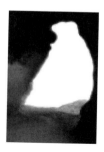

NEUTRAL ZONE

A gain, we were in Eulogio's room, by his *chiminea*. The fire soothed us both. Its flickering light allowed a peaceful, yet exhilarating flow of feelings. After a few delicious moments of silence, Eulogio began to speak.

"One thing that you should become increasingly aware of is the neutral zone," he said. "This is the core of what Esmeralda, Huang, and I are teaching you. That neutral zone, or place between our learned behaviors, is where the spirit grows and takes new form. Through it we allow ourselves to make new contact with the world."

He leaned back and slipped into the soothing sound of the fire.

"What have you been doing with Esmeralda lately?" he asked.

I recounted the ritual in the bullring. I added that somehow my perception of people had changed after that experience. I also noticed that I had more energy in my life as a whole.

"What Esmeralda was showing you in this ritual was that, first of all, you have to have realizations. Realizations are a form of gathering energy. Then, you need to integrate them into your body.

"If you're full of realization, and it's not spread throughout the body, so-called 'Zen sicknesses' can occur. Zen sicknesses appear when you expand too quickly and don't integrate the energy through the physical body, out through the relating body, and beyond. If you keep feeding your inner fire, and don't develop a way of expressing and stabilizing it in your body and in the world, a congestion or sickness can result. Such congestions cannot be remedied with medicines, because they are diseases of the spirit. They are beyond any consensual form of medicine because they deal with energies that are beyond the parameters of the consensual idea of the body of the time in which we live."

"Why can't medicine fix these diseases?" I asked, intrigued.

"Consensual medicine," he answered, "whether it is from the East or the West, is based on a consensual idea of the body—a common belief of what the body is and how to patch it up and keep it going on the same track.

"When one moves beyond this idea, medicine doesn't work anymore.

"What you have to realize is that medicine is created to keep the consensus alive, to perpetuate the consensual view—in Esmeralda's terms, the current male-female agreement. As a result, consensual medicine will support the limited societal view of what we are as humans and fight vehemently against anything that does not support this view. Remember, society is involved in trying to perpetuate itself, not in expanding the awareness of what is human.

"When one's idea of one's self and one's body moves beyond this view, a new fluid medicine is required."

He paused reflectively for a moment.

"There is little that has meaning for me anymore besides feeling the spirit move," Eulogio said. "Sickness often provides a door for the spirit to move through. That is one reason I enjoy this work. I come across people at an important juncture, and I have the opportunity to watch and even help the spirit move." As he said this, he filled with brilliance.

He sipped his tea, watched the fire, and then went on. "We lost much of our awareness and the necessary pressure to maintain it, by focusing all of our energy into our social contracts. The people I see need to learn to refocus their attention away from the male-female agreement and the social contracts.

"This is so easy and yet so hard," he said, chuckling.

"They need to learn to become a conduit for the spirit. They can then regain the innate confidence of the spider just beginning its web."

Eulogio paused for a moment and looked at the shadows on the wall.

"In the midst of one's learned behavior, one has to relax and stay neutral," Eulogio continued.

"That means you are neither reacting for nor against the learned behavior. It takes a great deal of energy to not respond, to be natural. This ability grows slowly. It has to be cultivated.

"When people's shields have been haphazardly rent," Eulogio went on, "the internal recognition of their innate being begins to become conscious, but their bodies and ways of relating cannot take the pressure of this new awareness. So neutrality has to be cultivated and then pitted against the electromagnetic patterns. We need to develop a strategy to give neutrality direction in the midst of our learned behavior.

"Learning to stay neutral in the midst of conditions provides a place where the spirit can grow without completely ripping apart the male-female agreement and the social contract. You can even learn to be neutral in the area of self and other, for here too there is a danger of getting distracted and allowing your idea of yourself to crystallize, to the exclusion of the motion of the spirit.

"The study of who we are is the study of motion. The neutral zone is the place of motion without motion, the In-Between."

This brought back the memory of what Esmeralda had put me through so that I could discover the observer in the midst of the four motions.

I told this to Eulogio.

He smiled knowingly and said, "The observer is the doorway to neutrality."

He sipped his tea and then continued.

"Learning not to react is also useful in dealing with illness. This is what healing is really all about."

"An attitude of neutrality allows one to move out of the way so that emotional reactions do not impede the body's natural healing process," he said. "For those whose shields have been rent and who suffer diseases because of that, it offers them a place from which to create a new world."

Eulogio leaned over and stirred the fire back to life, using a special stick that he had next to the *chiminea*. "Fire doesn't like to be touched by metal. Touch it with wood. Fire likes that better."

He put a couple of logs on the fire, then sat back.

"In terms of the body, the patterns we have learned constrict the ways that we move," he said. "This repetitious, nonvarying way of moving begins to wear the body out and take away its spontaneity. The luminous cell begins to crinkle up and lose its tone."

He reached over to his paper pile, picked up a paper sack, and crinkled it.

"When you become neutral and relax, you begin to build pressure. Relaxing builds pressure. You start to open up from within, and this is where true gains are made. Neutrality, or emptiness, creates a situation where new and unexpected variations of behavior or motion are created.

"Here, acupuncture can be helpful," he said, "because it can place the body in a neutral zone, for a while, where previously constricted body energies can flow."

Eulogio paused to stare at the fire for a moment.

"If we look at Michelle," he continued, "we can see how her beliefs create a structure throughout her body which predisposes her to certain types of disease."

I told Eulogio that I still wasn't clear about what he meant.

"She has been taught to act a certain way, in this case 'the beautiful woman,' and this gets supported by her surrounding cast—parents, family, both men and women," he said. "She is very confined in her contact with the world at large. The limitation that her body feels is directly related to the male-female agreement of this time. She is a superb expression of what it epitomizes.

"What we see graphically, in her case," he continued, "is that the seat of her problems is in her lower abdomen. The male-female agreement limits what she is allowed to play out in this area. From there, crinkles or interconnected bands of tightness manifest up and down the body, causing various diseases.

"We'll talk about this more specifically tomorrow morning. For now, remember what I told you earlier about the importance of treating the major pattern first, and then fitting the symptoms into it? The major pattern in Michelle comes from this area below the navel. This is true for all people, but Michelle is an especially graphic example.

"Loosening the binding places that hold Michelle so tightly, with acupuncture, for example, allows her to relax into the integrity of her body and physically enables her to experience neutrality," he said.

"Neutrality is just relaxing, not relating to the world from the perspective of learned behavior," he continued. "It's acting from a third place, neither for nor against the old patterns. This is really the only way for her to make progress or go beyond her learned behavior."

"Does this mean she has to become a nun?" I asked.

Eulogio looked at me and laughed.

"If Michelle were constantly to negate her attractiveness," he said, "she would reinforce her patterns as much as if she were actively involved in putting them forward.

"What is important is for her to move away from her frame of reference and observe herself from another position. The difficulty that she experiences is that she has spent a great deal of time in her learned behavior and is afraid of letting it go."

Eulogio once again picked up his stick and stirred the fire. He sat back, looked at me, and continued.

"When she is relaxing into neutrality, she can gather some of the energy that she usually expends supporting her old behavior patterns and allow something greater, the spirit, to redirect it. It is very difficult for her, primarily because it is the first step. It is the first time she has tried to be neutral in the midst of conditions," he said.

"In the short run, it is necessary to treat her symptoms to alleviate the pain," he continued, "but without a constant emphasis on the real problem—the male-female agreement—the symptoms will just shift around. Remember that the crinkles go up and down her luminous cell so that she can have a dysfunction anywhere along them.

"It is also important to extend the new awareness that we create through treatments in her physical body to her relating body," he said. "So, I give her exercises to do in her relating body. These are to allow this new awareness to interact in the world. I give her specific tasks that will disrupt her usual way of relating and thus create a pause, a kind of neutrality, a space in her way of relating that begins to allow for spontaneity to surface."

Eulogio leaned back, stretched for a minute, and continued.

"Don't expect to digest all this at once," he said. "But somewhere you will store this knowledge, and it will surface at the appropriate time. That is the way bodies talk to bodies."

Eulogio made motions with his hands as if they were mouths talking to each other, like we did when we were children. He chuckled.

He looked over at me, then continued.

"I think it's really important for you to understand how we are walled in by fears which keep us in our learned patterns."

I thought about my experience in the bullring and was able to see that the body plate which I was attempting to move away from had been created by fear.

"The way in which we are bound by fear becomes clear when we try and loosen the grip of our old patterns," Eulogio continued.

"There are two fears that arise when we start to disrupt our old ways, and these fears are very real," he said. "One is the fear and paranoia of not being able to maintain the social contracts we have been taught. This is a fear of being excommunicated from the system, the only system we know.

"There is also the very real fear of our aloneness. This is a fear of not having the energy to face the pressure that the world at large will exert on us if we give up the learned behavior into which we have put all our energy."

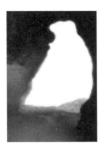

LUMINOUS BODY

T he next morning we rose early. It was my last day with Eulogio, and he wanted to show me something at the clinic. Walking to the office at this early hour was different. There were many birds singing in the trees. There weren't as many people out.

With the slight hint of winter chill in the air, we walked more quickly than usual. When we got to the clinic it was quiet for the first time since I had been there. There was a good feeling to the place that I hadn't noticed amidst all of the usual activity.

Eulogio led me into his office and sat down behind his desk. He motioned for me to have a seat.

He pointed to a triptych hanging on his wall. The center panel was an antique Tibetan painting of a yogi whose entire torso, arms, and legs were visible. Inside the trunk of the figure three lines had been drawn from the perineum to the crown of the head and down over the forehead. The center line was blue, there was a red line on the right, and a white line on the left. At intervals the lines on the sides looped around the center line and back again, constricting the central line and forming knots where they intersected along the mid-line.

"The blue line in the center," Eulogio said, "represents our true nature, our divine possibility. Buddhists would call it the Buddha-nature. I've been talking to you about it in terms of the place of neutrality, where our natural spontaneity exists. The white and red lines form knots of duality around it. The knots constrict this true nature and siphon its energy off in specific ways, depending upon which part of the body the knot resides in.

"The task of the ancient yogi was to loosen these knots, so that his Buddha-nature could merge with the world through his body. Or, so that his idea of his body could become so elastic that it would allow for the waves of universal energy to move through him."

Eulogio then pointed to the picture on the left. It was the same sort of figure, only in this one, the knots had been elaborated into many-petaled flowers with Sanskrit letters in their centers.

"In this picture the particular ways the knots have been tied around our true nature have been developed into centers called *chakras*. The ways that the knots are tied begin to take forms that have some sense of tangibility. Many people talk about *chakras* without realizing that they come from this other picture," he said, pointing back to the central picture in the triptych. "They value the energy that is gathered there. They don't realize that the *chakras* are formed through a constriction of our true energy. The aim is not to intensify the pattern that is centered there, but to dissolve the duality that created them—to untie the knots."

He turned to the picture on the right, which was also a forward-facing figure. It had colored circles bearing Sanskrit letters at the positions of the *chakras*, and superimposed lines showing the acupuncture meridians.

"The *chakras* are formed, and the energy is carried out to these meridians that you see," he said. "I am sure that Huang has already told you that the meridians are the rivers of energy and light that flow in the connective tissue.

"This idea of connective tissue is a concept out of Western anatomy and physiology. We use it because it seems to fit. Using this idea of connective tissue can be a doorway, we believe, to a multisensual view of the body. This view is more complete than the restricted mental-visual view of the body popular in the West today."

He stopped and looked out the window. "It isn't that the Western viewpoint is bad, but its variables of perception are limited and incomplete. More specifically, it lacks an idea of the purpose or potential of the human form. Thus it lacks a sense of direction."

I was puzzled. I confessed this to Eulogio.

"I went off on a tangent," Eulogio chuckled, "Let's get back to our drawings."

He smiled, and turned back to look at the triptych again. He began pointing and explaining.

"We are first undifferentiated energy that knows all. That energy or spirit becomes bound by duality by the two side channels as they form the *chakras*. The energy flows from there, out the twelve main meridian pathways—the rivers in the connective tissue—where it is shaped into our idea of the body.

"The connective tissue is bound into patterns," he said. "More specifically, the male-female agreement and the resultant social contracts actually reside in the patterns of binding in the connective tissue.

"You *comprende?*" he said, rapping me on the head with his knuckles, and laughing.

I looked up, giving him my total attention.

"The central channel," he continued, "is what Esmeralda has described to you as the light in the middle of our being, shining out through our idea of the body into the world. She also told you how learned behavior limits what you perceive. Patterns are created in the connective tissue that crinkle up your luminous membrane."

He stopped and looked at me.

"What she did not tell you was that there is a template or a knowledge of how the spirit can merge with the world at large.

"This template is the proper way for the web of light to shine through your physical form. It can be felt as a part of you that knows how you should be, running from the central core of your being to the most distant part of yourself. This template gives us the form we are trying to grow into. And, at the same time, its very existence makes us want to grow into it.

"On a physical level, the template is what heals the body," he said. "Truly healing a physical illness is moving into more direct contact with this template."

Eulogio then rubbed his chin as if he was pulling on an imaginary goatee.

"Looking at life from this primordial idea of the body," he said, "sickness is a process through which our body of knowledge is trying to reconnect itself with the world at large. Sickness is the spirit's way of trying to work through misinformation, trying to work through an erroneous sense of duality which separates this primordial idea of the body from its true expression in the world. Sickness, from this perspective, can be seen as a signal that tells us that a certain way of interacting with the world has worn out and that our luminous essence is looking for new expression.

"Let's see this in a more practical light," Eulogio said. "Let's look at someone like Michelle.

"If someone is an ideal of the male-female agreement of the time, like a very beautiful woman, that person is subjected to strong pressures from both within and without to maintain a specific and very rigid way of being. From the inside, Michelle feels that she can get her needs met very easily. She needs to exert very little energy, and in only a few limited ways, to obtain whatever she wants from the social contract. From the outside, there is a pressure exerted by the collective learned behavior. This learned behavior has a lot invested in making sure that someone who expresses its ideals behaves the way she is expected to."

He looked at me and raised his eyebrows.

"People who epitomize the ideals, such as beautiful women, are under a lot of pressure from the outside, and from the inside, so they see little reason to change or to explore anything new," he continued.

His words allowed me to see how acculturated I was and made me realize what a monumental task it was to free myself from my learned behavior.

"The knots in which the male-female agreement tie these 'perfect people' will be rigid and tight," he said. "They will have few variations in the ways that they can contact the world. The constant repetition of interacting along these limited lines of expression will lead to constriction of the connective tissue in the genital area, and from there, throughout the body."

Eulogio turned to face me.

"Right here at the navel center is where we receive nourishment when we are in the womb." Eulogio pointed to his belly.

"This is where we still receive nourishment. During digestion, this is the center where we process food and nourish ourselves, just as if we had an umbilical cord. Psycho-emotionally, this is where we receive vibrations and inputs and interchanges from the world around us. It is where we learn to differentiate our learned idea of the body from all of the other possibilities available to us. Both physically and psycho-emotionally, the navel is the seat of our learned behavior."

Eulogio began rubbing his belly. He looked up at me with an impish grin and began giggling.

"From the navel upwards are what the Chinese call the celestial energies," he continued. "From the navel downwards exist the earthly energies, specifically those of sexuality, defecation, and urination. It is in this latter area that the creative forces reside and, from there, flow through the rest of the body.

"These lower energies are what social structures try to contain," he said, purposely smiling the contained, frozen smile which I'd often observed on a politician or a homecoming queen.

"In their attempts to restrain and direct these energies," he went on, "these structures severely limit the expression of the body's creative forces. This limitation means that certain aspects of ourselves are overused, and others not used at all, creating what we have called 'crinkles' in the connective tissue. This plasters the connective tissue together, so that areas of the body interact like rigid blocks instead of having fluid motion."

He stopped momentarily, then continued.

"Making this area below the navel into a block limits the fluidity there. This then causes diseases throughout the body.

"As the male-female agreement is the root of the social contracts, constriction in the genital area is the origin of diseases that run up and down the body.

Eulogio had me fascinated. He was able to touch on many of

the feelings I had experienced and blend them with the medical knowledge I had learned.

"What I want you to hear is that the male-female agreement of the times, and the diseases that we experience in our bodies, whether in the physical or relating body, are one and the same thing," he said. "Seeing this is what will help you to understand how diseases in all different parts of the body are expressions of the same imbalance that begins with the male-female agreement in the genital area."

"So we are stuck on the physical level, too," I said, realizing that I had even more to deal with than I had originally thought. I again was struck by the implications of the all-encompassing nature of our learned behavior.

"So how do we grow beyond our learned behavior?" I asked.

"In general, the key to releasing the constrictions of the connective tissue is allowing the healing body, our innate nature, to express itself," he said.

"The way to do this in the relating body is by acting neutrally. In the physical body, it is learning to relax and create pressure. This allows the spirit to flow through the body."

Eulogio stopped talking. He relaxed for a moment. He then had me sit back in my chair and relax. He directed me to look at the triptych. He told me to let my eyes unfocus so that I could see all three of the images at once. He said that this was a magical picture if looked at in the right way.

As I unfocused my eyes on the picture, he placed one hand at the base of my skull and the other on top of my head, pressing gently.

Suddenly, instead of three pictures, I saw one. This picture was alive and moved. I saw a central channel constricted by knots which formed flowers with many petals. From the tip of each petal, red and white lines issued out to form into the shape of a body. As I kept concentrating, the central channel stood out and blue lines emanated from it, forming another body superimposed on the first. The red and white lines dissolved and, finally, there was just a picture of a pulsating human form made of blue lines emanating from the central core.

From the image before me, I experienced the realization that there is a volition body, a healing body, and a body of true knowledge. At that moment, I knew that it was possible for me to transcend my learned behavior and become something greater. I knew that it was possible to embody the spirit in the human form, and more.

I heard Eulogio's voice, very softly and intensely. "There is something in us that knows," he said.

He released my head and sat in his chair. The image dissolved. I turned around to look at him. He looked radiant. He leaned over, patted me on the shoulder, and laughed.

After a few moments, he turned to a figure on an anatomical chart. He pointed to the genital area. "When this area has pressure and is strong, the rest of the body is strong and interconnected.

"Our learned behavior has the effect of disrupting the interconnectedness of the body. Because of this, we lose pressure," he continued.

"When we begin to learn the male-female agreements and social contracts of our time, the connective tissue becomes plastered together into blocks. This blocking constricts the flow of energy between the lower body and the upper body. A separation begins to occur between the earthly energies and the celestial energies at the level of the navel," he said as he pointed back and forth, above and below the navel.

"The engine that runs the body is here, in the abdomen," he said, pointing to the navel area.

"When the learned behavior plasters together the connective tissue into blocks, the ability of this area to feed the rest of the body becomes limited. At the same time, the reciprocal relationship between this part of the body and the rest is lessened. The interconnectedness of the whole body is diminished."

He paused for a moment, then continued.

"The end result is that, in terms of energy, the ribcage separates from the abdomen. All diseases come essentially from this separation. The Chinese say that the top part of the torso is yang, and the bottom part is yin, and that when yin and yang separate, you die."

Eulogio then showed me, through the anatomical and acupuncture charts on the walls of his office, how disruptions in the genital system cause problems in other parts of the body.

"For example, in women," he said, "a problem in the genital area can cause problems directly in the breast and throat. The bowels, which are in proximity to the genital area, also begin to suffer." He went on to explain how constrictions in the lower abdominal area lead to problems in both men and women.

He explained how loosening up the flow of the acupuncture meridians, or the flow of energy through the connective tissue using acupuncture needles, could help these problems.

He went on to say that seeing the genital area as the seat of energy in the body, and its lack of flow as the cause of illness, would allow me to understand disease much more clearly. Then, I would be able to look at the body and understand how seemingly unrelated sets of symptoms could be seen as ramifications of the same pattern.

He stopped for a moment. There was a knock on the door. One of his students had arrived, along with Eulogio's first patient of the day.

Suddenly the serious, erudite man that I had known changed into a charming, courteous joker with a jukebox-full of bizarre songs at his disposal and buttons just waiting to be pressed.

He looked at me with a twinkle in his eye and said, "Say hello to all those old folks up there!"

He gave me a light handshake, chuckled, and said in a confidential tone, "Don't forget!"

Then, as he waved good-bye, he leaned toward me and sang in a deep, throaty voice, "Don't try and run all night, don't try and run all day, don't bet your money on a bobtail nag, oh doo-dah day!"

PART FIVE

TRUSTING THE BODY

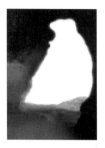

THE PROCESS

After my visit with Eulogio, I headed back north in my truck. As I drove, I thought about the early spring in the high desert where I lived. It was my least favorite season. Not only was I forced to wake up from the stillness and introspection of winter, but I had to do it in the most jarring of fashions. Beautiful sunshine one day, wind the next, snow and rain interspersed—not to mention mud. The scurrying frenzy of new projects bursting forth carried me along like a rushing stream that led only to greater and greater turbulence.

Each year I became a little more used to it. I surrendered more easily to the process of the change of seasons.

As I drove, I thought about the knowledge that Eulogio had shared with me. In retrospect, I saw that what he had reiterated in so many different ways was that we are a process, a movement, and that by being neutral, we could allow our process to flow until, eventually, we could become the process itself.

When we identify ourselves with this process, rather than with who we think we are or how we think we should act, we begin a cycle of continual renewal, which catapults us into a magical new world that is recreated for us every moment.

I leaned over and grabbed a bottle of water and looked out at the expanse of sky all around me.

Thinking again about Eulogio, I recalled what he told me about volition. He had said that volition works out from the center of our being, through the physical body, through the relating body, and out to the world beyond. He said that the spirit works through the body to disrupt our old ways of being in order to allow us new options and more contact with the world.

He went on to say that, as people, we are very slow and don't let go of our old patterns until we absolutely have no other choice. Sickness in the physical body, or life situations in the relating body, provide the pressure to make this happen.

Trusting our basic instinct, relaxing and becoming our process, is what we have to learn. Underneath the turmoil that we perceive as ourselves, there is a stability and a force that supports us.

These thoughts reminded me of the last time I was with Michelle, when I had talked to her for a short time in one of Eulogio's treatment rooms.

Michelle had come into Eulogio's clinic that day distraught and confused. She had pain in her jaw and a headache and complained of a host of other maladies throughout her body.

She said that she had done some of the things Eulogio had told her to do at home with her family and had gotten an intensely hostile reaction. I then remembered Eulogio telling me that, when you first begin to face your fears, you are struck the hardest.

I noticed how contracted Michelle had become. It was clear to me that facing her fears had brought on this reaction.

Eulogio had walked in with a smile. He asked her a few simple questions and then placed some needles in her body. He remained in the room and continued to talk to her. I noticed a remarkable shift in the room as Michelle's energy changed. From the state of confusion and contraction she had been in, she quickly became another person, and a much fuller communication was possible between all of us.

Eulogio told her a couple of off-color jokes, and she began to laugh. He then gave her an explanation of the change that she had just gone through. He talked at length about how she had changed from a state of contraction, full of pain, to another in which she felt open and connected. He said it was important for her to remember that this kind of change was possible. He encouraged her to remember, as well as she could, the stages that she had gone through which allowed it to happen.

Eulogio told her that right after she had gone through this process of transformation was an important time to pause and reflect. This would give her body a chance to digest what she had learned, and that even if her mind didn't remember, her body would.

I remembered Eulogio saying that we have to go over and over things countless times before they sink in and we can remember them. And we have to go over them countless times more before we can learn how to act with this new knowledge we have gained.

He said that his role was to help make her more conscious of the pathway and that stopping to acknowledge what has happened helps this knowledge sink in more quickly.

He went on to say that another one of his functions was to provide her with a living model—himself—to show her that real change was possible.

A new vocabulary, he had said, begins to develop in our being in which motions which were inexpressible before become accessible. As this vocabulary moves through the relating body, it strengthens and stabilizes new ways of contacting the world.

I chuckled to myself as I drove, remembering the many confusions I had gone through trying to understand who Eulogio, Huang, or Esmeralda were talking to or what they were laughing at.

Then I went back to thinking about Eulogio and Michelle.

After he had left the room, Michelle asked me about what he had said. I had told her about my experiences of falling apart with Esmeralda. They had been very painful for me but, having gone through them, I now had to agree with what Eulogio had said.

I told Michelle that I was thankful to her and to the spirit for allowing me to witness her process of falling apart. It made a feeling of completion for me.

We laughed together, wondering what Eulogio would say about this. Eulogio marched in as if on cue. He began telling Michelle that it was important to learn how to fall apart and come back together. This process is the spirit in action, he had said. It is much like the pressure that a flower bud feels as it opens, painful on the inside and beautiful on the outside. Eulogio laughed and said to both Michelle and me, "It must appear to be such a paradox to you now."

He said that this is the process of learning to identify with one's own nature, and not with the forms that it takes. "It's like identifying the nature of the water apart from the waterfall, or the slow-flowing river, or the ocean waves."

Thinking about this, I began to feel disoriented. It seemed I was driving very slowly. However, when I looked down at the speedometer, I realized that I was doing eighty-five. So I slowed down a little.

As I drove on, I began remembering more of what Eulogio had told Michelle. He had told her that diseases and the demands one feels from one's family and friends are related. They are obstacles or confusions that one must penetrate.

Eulogio had said that you do this by staying neutral and relaxing. You need to meet these obstacles and confusions with patience, pressure, and concentration. In this way, you can undo a disease or ignorant way of thinking about the body.

He went on to say that, when you first begin to allow your process of renewal to flow through you, you are hit the hardest by the pressures that formed your idea of the body. Because you don't yet have the strength to relax into your process, you don't yet recognize what your process is, so you have no confidence in it.

I recalled that later I had asked Eulogio why he had talked to Michelle for so long about such abstract subjects. He replied that she had shifted and, in her new state of awareness, it wasn't hard for her to understand him.

He went on to say that this shift was the opportunity he had been waiting for. Her being was much more integrated in this new state, so that she had the pressure and strength to understand what he told her. He wanted to keep her there, in that state, and he had used descriptive words to stabilize it and give it context.

He said that words can serve as a way to remember a certain new state of mind. He wanted Michelle to examine that state, to log in hours there, and to feel the new landscape inside of her being, so that it could become real to her mind and body.

As I drove, I relaxed my eyes. They began to unfocus, and I became aware of my peripheral vision. The view of the highway that I had been perceiving became less concrete. I no longer saw the same road. Instead, I saw the road with each of my eyes, rather than the one road I saw when focusing my eyes together. I felt disoriented. But I worked on maintaining this perception of two roads at once, using my peripheral vision. Much to my surprise, I found that I could still drive. At first, I didn't feel safe, but I got accustomed to this new perception.

As I maintained this view of the road, I was struck by something that Eulogio had said. "Your witnessing of Michelle's process makes a completion for you. This will allow you to fall apart more smoothly yourself.

"If you go through something, and then you turn around and look at what you went through by witnessing somebody else go through something similar, you can more clearly grasp your own process.

"This gives your process a context: two positions from which to view it. With two points, the process begins to have texture. You gain depth and dimension. You begin to see your own landscape more clearly, and have more confidence in your process."

I was nearing home. Soon I would resume my studies with Huang. What new perspective on my process would he offer now?

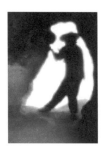

REFLEXIONES:
MY GROWTH THROUGH GRAVITY

Personally, the most healing thing that I have ever done has been to learn that gravity—the earth's force—is, in a very simple sense, the sustaining force of my physical presence here on earth. The more that I have been able to sink down into this primordial thought, trust it, and allow it to work through me, the fuller and more complete my life has become. This love that the earth has for me, and I for it, has taught me to see that my idea of the body was just that, an idea—a multisensual idea that I could explore and change.

The more efficient my idea of my body in its relationship to gravity and the resultant flow, the more dimensions I can experience with less stress on my being. I have come to realize that there is a very efficient way to walk on the earth and that, when I can maintain this fluid posture, I create a stable platform from which to explore and understand the meaning of why I am here. When the relationship between my idea of the body and gravity is maximized, I save energy and thus have more energy to achieve my potential. I call this learning the study of body mechanics.

Huang taught me about body mechanics by teaching me specific exercises that allowed me to feel and understand how the body works through its relationship to gravity and the result-ant pressure that is produced. These exercises were a very prac-tical way of retraining my body to align better with gravity and thus pump more energy through it.

The ramifications of this training in my personal life have been enormous. I have been able to create—at a very deep, sup-portive level—new points of focus outside my cultural matrix from which to deal with the world. As simple as this is to say, this new focus is difficult to experience, because I am talking about a way of being with our bodies that is beyond the linguistic and cultural framework with which we all grew up. In essence, it is about learn-ing to live in a different sensual mix—in a reality that is at the same time greater than but inclusive of our learned behavior.

For one thing, the abdomen became very important to me as an intersection between the inner and outer sides of ourselves. In Western culture, the importance of the abdomen has been hidden, and this discovery and its implications have done much to free me.

I've learned that if one can change the tone or loosen up the connective tissue in the abdomen, one can, in a very direct way, change one's emanation into the world and thus change one's life. In particular, because so much of our social condition-ing is based on society's fear and control of sexual energy, learn-ing to loosen the lower abdomen and pelvis has given me a great understanding of the underpinnings that hold us together as a culture yet limit our personal growth.

For me personally, these realizations about relaxing my ab-domen have given me cues of ways to act in social interactions, ways to begin breaking down my learned behavior. I began to see that when I interacted with people, I had a tendency to be static rather than moving with optimal gravitational flow. By learning to line up better with gravity and move more energy through my body, I was able to flow through a lot of my normal defense mechanisms and establish greater contact with the world at large. By focusing on my abdomen while in the midst of a social interaction, I could break down the patterns that had been stamped into me. As I stabilized these new ways of being, I have become more transparent and hide less from the world.

By studying internal martial arts—Chinese yoga and body mechanics, which are really the study of our relationship to gravity or the earth's force—I have been able to see how bodies talk to bodies and how we each have a different idea of our body. Through exercises, I gradually learned to have more contact with the world and other people by first having more contact with my body. This simplified my life and has allowed me to live with less clutter and more efficiency. As a result, my life has become fuller and richer.

Another change that I noticed was that I began to see that I could access meditative states, which I had previously experienced only in periods of sitting meditation, when moving my body alone or around other people. Essentially, what Huang taught me was to relax my body and keep it relaxed in the midst of motion. Thus, I was able to move off the mediation pillow into the world of people and flow in those situations. I saw that I had learned to relax in the midst of getting hit by the body-to-body cultural framework we all grew up with. I found that the new points of focus that I had sensually established allowed me to flow through situations in which I would normally have become a static object.

Finally, for many years I had been troubled by the theoretical inconsistencies that I noticed in the conventional study of acupuncture and Chinese medicine. Though I made my living by healing people using these methods, I often felt caught in a crossfire. I would read many books, but each espoused a different and often conflicting theory.

However, as my studies of body mechanics progressed, I came to realize that many of the people writing these books never experienced their bodies outside the context of the conventional idea of the body of the times in which they lived. Rather, they had read other books written by people who hadn't looked at their bodies either, until a tangential notion of the body was created.

But when I began at last to feel the textured, mulltisensual tapestry of my body, all the extrapolations and seeming contradictions started to clear up. Everything I read and everything that I had learned through my healing practice became relevant and simple. I understood in a new way how many diseases are caused by our social conditioning. This realization helped me devise better treatment strategies. I now function as a healer with more confidence.

Accepting gravity and the force of the earth as a teacher was what has put me on the path towards wholeness. I have learned from this wonderful source how our personal interactions, the way that we position ourselves, and our emotional makeup are linked to create our sense of well-being.

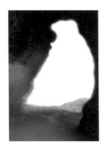

THINKING, FEELING, BEING

S pringtime for me, as usual, was complete chaos. New ideas, new projects, were sprouting to life with seeming abandon. Each one came to life in an undifferentiated profusion.

The only calm in the storm were my classes with Huang. They seemed to exist outside of time. When I stepped into his presence, my sense of time warped, and my memory became contextual instead of linear.

One day I was working with him in his studio. He had already shown me an exercise and was watching me practice. He reminded me, as he often did, to keep my shoulders and elbows down. This time, however, he gave me an explanation.

"When you press down on your shoulders and elbows properly, it reconnects your ribcage back with your abdomen." I stopped the exercise in order to listen to him.

"Keep moving!" he said. I want you to feel this as I talk, and I want you to put it in your body."

I began doing the exercise again. He moved to my side, and continued to talk. He touched my chest.

"This is where all your vital organs are kept. Your heart, your lungs, your spleen, your liver, and your kidneys, are all protected by your ribcage."

He placed his hand on my abdomen.

"This is where your working organs are housed. They are called your yang organs in Oriental medicine. They do the work. They interact with the world. If you make this area strong you become more resilient.

"This is where the cooking takes place—the Great Cauldron. Here is where your hollow organs are, where actual processing and pressure-cooking goes on. Food goes through the stomach, the small intestine, and the large intestine like going through a big snake. All the way through the snake it gets pressurized and processed. Leftover solids come out the rectum, and liquids out the bladder."

He stepped back and watched me for a while. Then he came closer and touched my head. "Thinking. All the internal chatter."

He then touched my chest. "Feeling. The emotions."

He touched my abdomen and said, "Being, the hub of it all."

He placed his hand on my face and forehead. "Remember, this is the screen that pulls up information from the computer."

He brushed his fingers lightly up and down my torso. He then placed his hands at the bottom of my ribcage, and said, "As our learned behavior takes hold of us, the ribcage begins to separate from the abdomen.

"Our work is to reunite the head, or the little thinking mind, with the chest, where the emotions are housed. Then we learn to reunite the chest area with the abdomen, where our sense of beingness resides. When we can unite these three parts of ourselves, we feel whole."

I lost my concentration.

"Don't think!" he said. "Experience. Keep moving. It's all coming together for you as we talk. Trust your body. Unite your body. You can't be aware of your whole body if you are caught up in thinking or your emotions."

He told me to move very slowly and deliberately. He wanted me to notice the complicated patterns of touching that I moved through. He told me to notice how my awareness could ripple through my body, sparking a series of sensations that were well beyond my ability to think or to grasp while in an emotional state.

I began to feel a rippling through my body. I felt multisensual currents flowing. As my awareness expanded, my ideas about myself broke down. I opened up to a new sensual world. In this world of being, my senses of sight, sound, and touch united and separated with ease into an unlimited variation of patterns. Light poured into long-forgotten chambers in my being, and I opened myself up to remembering who I was.

Huang kept a sharp eye on me. Like the proctor in a Zen meditation, whenever I began to think, he would make contact with me, either using his hand to correct some movement or reminding me verbally to concentrate.

"You have to stay in this state of being long enough to build a memory," Huang said.

After I had been practicing this exercise for quite a while, Huang stood in front of me and began to do the complementary movements to the exercise that he had just taught me. He made light contact with me. When my body moved forward, his moved back, and when his moved forward, mine moved back.

Soon after we started, I lost the awareness that I had felt when doing the exercise on my own.

He stopped me. "Up until now, you've been borrowing energy from me when we move together. Today, I want your strength to come from your own sense of self."

He initiated our movement again and kept talking as we moved. "Feel the way that you were feeling while doing the exercise by yourself. I want you to feel that same strength, as if I were not here making contact with you."

I tried to recapture the feeling that I had had when I was moving alone. It was difficult for me with another person so close. I kept thinking, wondering if I was doing the movement right, trying to correct myself, and feeling uncomfortable.

Suddenly I found myself flying across the room. Huang smiled and said, "Thinking a lot, aren't you? Let's try it again."

We began moving together again. I not only kept trying to correct myself but was apprehensive about the possibility of once again being thrown across the room. What he did to me never seemed to hurt. He was always in control. It just shocked me for a few seconds.

It wasn't long before I was airborne again. Time stood still. I didn't know how to act. I lost my idea of who I was. I was afraid to be in that exposed state of just being with another person. I felt I needed my habitual patterns to defend myself, but the second I pulled myself back together in the old way, I would be sent flying.

Finally Huang put his hands down and crossed his arms. He looked at me intently with a smile on his face and said, "Don't go back to your obsessions. That's not the way to put yourself back together. Stay connected to your abdomen.

"First I wanted you to experience this feeling of connectedness by yourself. The next step is to ground it into your being by relating in this new way to another person. It's difficult to maintain this feeling during interactions with others. It requires more concentration and pressure than maintaining it when you are alone.

"Your old patterns are more easily triggered when I am close to you than when you are doing an exercise alone. Learning how to be in close with someone else, yet staying relaxed and flowing as if you were concentrating alone, is what we are after. There are many feelings we can have when we are alone, but they don't really become useful or stabilized until they can be done around other people. So let's try it again. This time I'll soothe you with my voice."

We began moving slowly again. Each time I began to wander, Huang would remind me to come back, at first with his voice and later simply by increasing the pressure on our point of contact. His body could read mine so well that the slightest lack of concentration on my part was quite apparent to him.

I still felt very inept at this new language he was teaching me. But, the overall effect it had on my life and my sense of well-being was unquestionable.

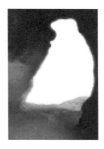

FLUIDITY

I left class that day and, instead of going home, went to a park near where I lived. I wanted to digest what I had learned. Huang always encouraged me to practice on my own. He told me I had to incorporate the teachings into my body until I could experience them without him.

As I practiced the movements that I had learned, I observed how my body changed as I became involved with either thoughts or emotions.

Eventually I began to see how my idea of the body changed when I was thinking, when I reacted emotionally, or when I was simply being. When I was thinking, I could not move my body nearly as smoothly, quickly, or interconnectedly as I could when I was just being. But when I was just being, I did not have to give up my center of thinking. I simply refused to allow my thoughts to control or obliterate my other sensations. In essence, I was keeping a guardian by an open gate, so that the power of thought was at my disposal but not in control.

I had to build up a great deal of energy in order to keep my concentration without letting it transform into thoughts. I felt like I was building an internal muscle.

I then looked at my emotions. In many ways, they were a stronger diversion than my thoughts. I had to learn to keep this center open, too, and set up a guardian at that gate. When I did this, it seemed to open up a way to the center of being in my abdomen, allowing me to feel whole.

At this point I realized that I was using the techniques that Huang had taught me to push my ribcage back into my abdomen. Doing this, I experienced a feeling of wholeness. In just allowing gravity to push the diaphragm and abdomen together, I was able to feel complete. It was so simple.

As I walked back to my truck, I remembered some lines of Chuang Tzu that Huang had once read to me.

> The breath of the true man rose up from his heels
> while the breath of common men rises from their throats.
> When they are overcome,
> their words catch in their throats
> like vomit.
> As their lusts and desires deepen,
> their heavenly nature grows shallow.

Amid the flow of classes that spring, there was one in particular that showed me what Huang was doing to free me from the confinement of my old conceptions of my body. Here I experienced the pain and work one has to go through to bring one's naked state of being forward in the presence of another person.

Huang was showing me how to use my eyes. "When facing another person," he said, "one should look with 'angry eyes,' with the eyes of a tiger. It is the detached, cool look of a fighting cock, the look a cat has when it freezes its prey.

"This makes you strong," he said. "This makes you present. This charges your body with volition. It keeps you from being fooled by another person, or more importantly, by your thoughts of another person.

"Now let me see you do it."

I put on a hard look, like I was staring someone down in the street, and did a couple of movements.

Huang burst out laughing. "You've missed the point," he said. "Look inward with your eyes. Feel your eyes looking out from the *dan tien* in the navel area. Look at the world from that point. This tiger and cock stuff is just a poetic way of getting you there. And I can see it didn't work!"

"Well, what do you mean by looking inward to the *dan tien?*" I asked.

Huang went nimbly over to the bookshelf in his studio and pulled out his copy of the translated writings of Chuang Tzu. He read a poem that was written about 300 B.C.

THE FIGHTING COCK

Chi Hsing Tsu was a trainer of fighting
   cocks
For King Hsuan.
He was training a fine bird.
The King kept asking if the bird were
Ready for combat.
"Not yet," said the trainer.
"He is full of fire.
He is ready to pick a fight
with every other bird. He is vain and confident
Of his own strength."
After ten days, he answered again:
"Not yet. He flares up
When he hears another bird crow."
After ten more days:
"Not yet. He still gets
That angry look
And ruffles his feathers."
Again ten days:
The trainer said, "Now he is nearly
   ready.
When another bird crows, his eye
Does not even flicker.

He stands immobile
Like a cock of wood.
He is a mature fighter.
Other birds
Will take one look at him
And run."

Huang then began talking to me slowly and deliberately.

"How one gazes at an opponent, or the world, or one's true opponent, oneself, is very important. If our eyes flit around, trying to figure out what we're up against, we can never move fast enough to be there. When the world gazes at us, we must return that gaze from the core of our being.

"If an opponent gazes at you, do not be caught in his gaze or what he might be thinking. Look inward, and you will react properly.

"When you look inward, it doesn't mean you don't see anymore. You look from a different position, not one of figuring things out, but a place of being. Looking inward opens up a new way of seeing. It's a way of connecting your true nature to the world through your eyes. Eventually you can feel how your eyes look from the navel. You actually learn to feel with your eyes.

"When your eyes look from your *dan tien,* you transcend what was and what will be, and you become present. Such seeing cuts through your old ways of being."

He moved to stand in front of me. He gazed at me. I was like a bird, frozen by the stare of a cat.

"Look at me," he said, "as if you were looking at your own death."

I looked at him and swallowed. "Looking at my own death?"

"Yes," he replied. "When you can gaze at your true opponent, yourself, in this way, you go beyond death.

"Look at me," he said.

He then took the posture for one of the two-man exercises we did together and gestured for me to join him. We began moving, wrists lightly touching, gazing at each other in the way he had described. It was very difficult for me to maintain enough concentration to support the intensity of this cold stare. It took me to a vast, somewhat fore-boding place. I tried to break my gaze with him, but he nudged me to remain engaged.

All of a sudden I was afraid of the intensity I saw in Huang. What if he hit me with that force? I became almost paralyzed with fear.

Huang nudged me. As my concentration came back, I realized that the fear I was feeling was really of my own violence, my own energy, and that was even more frightening. I began lowering my hand to stop. Huang nudged me again and caught me in his gaze. We continued.

A surge of emotion came through me, and I began to weep. Tears streamed down my face. He encouraged me to continue gazing and moving. I was struggling to let myself flow with waves of energy of an intensity that I couldn't remember ever having felt. Then, as abruptly as it had come, the emotion disappeared. Somehow I felt strong and relaxed. The energy spread through my body. We continued a while longer until Huang decided to stop.

"What happened?" he asked.

I tried to explain to him as best I could that I had felt this energy, this violence, come up in me that I had always been afraid of and had never let surface. I told him that I first thought the violence was in him and then realized that it was the violence in me. Fear of my own violence was what I had been experiencing, and it had been almost more than I could take.

"It's very common to confuse violence with energy," Huang said. "You have not been taught to function with so much voltage, with this much fluidity. You are taught to function in stiff, confined ways. Using more voltage threatens those ways and is seen as violence, when it's really just opening up to a whole new world. The expression of energy is limited in our culture, so sex and violence stick out because they require a lot of energy."

He put his hands on his groin. "The seat of energy in the body is in the genital area. We are taught very few ways of expressing this energy, and those ways are very contained. When you begin func-tioning with a greater volume of energy, you must face your ideas of sex and violence. Both violence and sex are controlled or prohibited within our social contracts."

He placed both of his hands on his lower abdomen.

"So when we are gazing, we are looking sex, violence, and the male-female agreement right in the eye. It's like sitting on a big ball of energy and realizing that you can relax. You don't have to panic. You're connected to your life force. You learn to trust it and it takes care of you. It's what's been taking care of you anyway. You're just becoming conscious of it and uniting yourself with it."

He relaxed his hands at his side, and continued. "We need to create enough pressure in our body to sustain this level of contact and allow it to find new expression. You only saw this energy as violent because you didn't know what else to do with it.

"What you just achieved in maintaining your concentration while being hit by your learned behavior and learning to relax through it is the key to our work. The world is always trying to fix us into a pattern—make us into objects—to make us solid.

"The volition, the spirit, seeks to flow. The new idea of the body that you are being impregnated with is a body that moves and flows."

He again walked over to the bookshelf. He pulled out a book and began to read aloud.

He who knows how to live can walk abroad
Without fear of rhinoceros or tiger.
He will not be wounded in battle.
For in him rhinoceroses can find no place to thrust their horn,
Tigers no place to use their claws,
And weapons no place to pierce.
Why is this so?
Because he has no place for death to enter.

"Because no one is there," Huang said slowly, as he looked up and grinned.

He put back his copy of Lao Tzu's *Tao Te Ching*, and continued. "This new idea of the body that we are stabilizing is a body of flow, not of objects. We move around objects, we move through objects, but we don't become objects.

"We can't be hit if there is nothing to hit," he said, his eyes twinkling.

"What allows us to do this? More energy.

"Create yourself into what your true nature wants, not what the world wants you to be. Understand the flow of things and become it."

He smiled.

"Our external patterns of touching change. The great new variety of sensations that we then experience disassembles our body's idea of itself. We gather enough energy to explode the idea of the body that is being maintained by the four motions of our learned behavior.

"Until we move away from our fixed idea of our body and its programmed reactions no real change can be made. When we become action, rather than a thing being acted upon, there is nothing to threaten us. We have nothing to defend. We are fluid."

POSTSCRIPT

At our core, we are light, the light that impregnated our first cell and made it grow. Our body is made up of ribbons of light creating a template. We spread that magical awareness out everyday to create our world. We are a luminous essence. We have a pattern within us that embodies our total human potential: a body that knows.

However, when we come into the world we are taught an idea of our body. This idea of who we are supposed to be limits the expression of our body that knows. Rather than embodying our total human potential, we manifest ourselves in a limited idea of the body. When we do this, we can only spread our light through that small portion of our being.

Because we can only feel whole and complete when we embody our potential, we feel a need to bring our light back into proper circulation. To do this we must understand both personal and cultural patterns of ill health and how our negative experiences of life are stored in areas of our bodies. We must also understand the manner in which diseases are culturally transmitted through generations and the way in which we are imprisoned by the cultural matrix within which we are raised.

In order to regain our true identity, we must begin to understand how to reclaim the light that we squander every day. This process of embodying our luminous essence affects our entire being down to the cellular level. We need to change the whole manner in which we communicate and interact within our multisensual reality.

Esmeralda once explained this to me quite clearly. I had asked her if the world could be changed through politics. She answered me by saying, "The only real politics are the politics that go on between bodies. If the way that bodies talk to bodies doesn't change, nothing really changes."

Closely examining how bodies talk to bodies—the multisensual way that we communicate—and the limitations placed upon that communication by our linguistic and cultural training has greatly changed the way that I view healing in my clinic. Now I have a broader context within which to understand what my patients are going through. I also experience that there is a higher mechanism upon which we depend to create harmony in the body and in our whole being.

The body models provided by the teachings that I received from Esmeralda, Huang, shamanistic healing, and Chinese medicine have shown me that our idea of the body is just a pattern through which greater forces work. As a result of my experiences and the spiritual pressure ignited in me by my teachers, I have seen that we are a flow and that identifying ourselves as a flow or a process is healing. I have been forced to expand my idea of who I am and realize that within me there is a body that knows, a luminous essence that is liquid light.

Reclaiming our light will most certainly mean that we will live our lives with an intense richness that we never knew existed. We can create a new vocabulary of bodies talking to bodies. This will allow us to experience a new world of sound, feeling, and light.

What is this light?

I once asked Eulogio that very question and I remember his response distinctly.

He looked at me, smiling, and said, "Light is a very arbitrary way to talk about our essence. But since we, as people, are so visual, we talk about it what way. It's really more of a luminous, liquid feeling.

"It's not what we usually see on a TV screen, or in our mental

176

projections upon the world. This I call 'flat light.' Flat light is visual but not luminous or liquid. Liquid light is multisensual and all-embracing. It is a full, complete feeling."

I thought for a moment, then asked, "What is the practical value of living in this luminous essence, this liquid light?"

He looked at me, lifted his eyebrows, and said, "For one thing, you won't have any time for opinions."

He chuckled. "You will lose your idea of your self and the ideas you have about your body. You will live in a bigger world."

And when I asked him for his thoughts on the new computer experiments with virtual reality, he looked at me and laughed.

"Why try to recreate the body," he asked, "when we already have one? Why not use what we have? It's better anyway. Our bodies will always be more complete than anything which can be invented."

We live in a sea of sensual inputs. We start to become very aware of this sea when we move outside of our learned behavior. The practical question then arises: How do we navigate our potential?

At this particular time in history, we in the West are, on the one hand, very fortunate to have a cornucopia of techniques, therapies, and spiritual paths from which to choose. Yet, we are confused and thus impoverished by not having a way to navigate through this maze of information.

I have found that if we use the idea of our body as a common denominator—since it actually is the common denominator through which we experience everything—we then have a vocabulary through which to create a new fluid model of reality. What I am suggesting is that we use the body for gathering and storing information as we move from one discipline, therapy, or spiritual path to another. Then, we can tap into our luminous essence and learn to use the natural integrity that our body has with the world to give us a sense of direction. In other words, we can use our luminous essence as an internal compass to guide us on our journey as we navigate through the calm waters and stormy seas of our multidimensional experience.

In my second book, *The Pressure of Affection*, Esmeralda, Huang, and Eulogio continue the exploration of our luminous essence, providing practical information and further techniques for achieving our full potential in this multisensual world.

I hope that *reading Luminous Essence* has sparked realizations in you that will help weave together any frayed threads in the tapestry of truth within which you live.

QUEST BOOKS
are published by
The Theosophical Society in America
Wheaton, Illinois 60189-0270
a branch of a world organization
dedicated to the promotion of the unity of
humanity and the encouragement of the study of
religion, philosophy, and science, to the end that
we may better understand ourselves and our place in
the universe. The Society stands for complete
freedom of individual search and belief.
For further information about its activities,
write, call 1-800-669-1571, or consult its Web page:
http://www.theosophical.org

*The Theosophical Publishing House
is aided by the generous support of
THE KERN FOUNDATION,
a trust established by Herbert A. Kern
and dedicated to Theosophical education.*